# Diary of an Eating Disorder

# DIARY OF AN EATING DISORDER

*A Mother and Daughter Share
Their Healing Journey*

## Chelsea Browning Smith

*with comments from her mother,*
Beverly Runyon

TAYLOR TRADE PUBLISHING
*Lanham • New York • Oxford*

Published by Taylor Trade Publishing
An Imprint of the Rowman & Littlefield Publishing Group
4501 Forbes Blvd., Suite 200
Lanham, Maryland 20706

Distributed by National Book Network

Smith, Chelsea Browning.
    Diary of an eating disorder : a mother and daughter share their healing journey / Chelsea Browning Smith ; with perspectives from her mother, Beverly Runyon.
        p.    cm.
    ISBN 0-87833-971-X
    1. Smith, Chelsea Browning—Mental health. 2. Eating disorders in adolescence—Patients—Biography. 3. Mothers and daughters.
4. Runyon, Beverly Browning—Diaries. I. Runyon, Beverly Browning.
II. Title.
RJ506.E18S64    1998
362.1'968526—dc21
[B]                                                                    98–9970
                                                                        CIP

Printed in the United States of America

To all those who lived these times with me. I give my journal to all the women and girls who know days like these and can call them their own.

# Contents

# Acknowledgments

I am forever thankful for my large family, who each had the courage to see, and ultimately hear the truth.

John Holt, my brother and first reader, who always insisted I believe. My time with you is never enough. My mom, for meeting and conquering your greatest fears, and even more, for having the courage to live your own life. You've given me the most unconditional love I've known. I love you both beyond reckoning.

Bill, who consistently loved and raised me as though I were his own. Keep climbing your mountains!

My dad, who taught me "there is nothing more powerful than the truth." Despite our distance I never doubted your love for me.

For all the laughter, energy, love, and continuous fun, I want to thank my best friends in the world. You will always remind me there is nothing more precious than life.

Jason Rath, my editor, for your calm and encouraging voice. Thank you for all your support.

Finally, Remuda, for the tools to fly! Dr. Don, Amy, the nurses, the Kellers, and all the women who walked with me in the darkest time of our lives. Thank you is never enough.

# Prologue

Every time I leave one of my sessions I feel better. We talk about stuff; I feel, express, and even cry. Today was the third time since I left her office to come home and throw up. I think things are getting better despite the fact that my mind focuses eighty percent of the time on food during the fifty-five minutes. But it's like the kitchen is a refuge for my mind. I always know it will be there, waiting to embrace me when I get home.

Alone is how I hope to find it. I have been thinking of what I will sink my teeth into first. Usually I go for the fat-free chocolate cake, then to the frozen yogurt, back to some bagel, and then finish with the frozen yogurt (which makes it all come up much smoother). I don't think this is normal, though I am not really concerned. I feel like a million-pound weight has been swept away by the effortless flush of the toilet. The hardest thing is to look in the mirror after I have thrown up. Sometimes I wipe my face before I look. Other times I leave the spit, bile, and food on my mouth and hands. I just stand there holding my hands up, with my shoulders slumped over. I produce this expression of absolute helplessness—then I laugh. I guess I am amazed by the act I've just committed. I can't explain why, I can't believe that it is really me doing this. Why would I do something like throw up? I really have no reason to torture myself. Bulimia was always *them*—I can't possibly be like that. I throw up, but I am not a bulimic. I sure as hell don't have an eating disorder.

I am totally for this whole counseling thing because I feel sad a lot and I want to feel better. But I can't leave there and not feel that I have to get this crap out. All this stuff that we talk about.

Today, Dr. Tant asked me when this all began. My first thought was, "Oh this throwing up thing? I really can't remember." But I do recall one time when my ex-boyfriend Matt and I had gone to a really nice dinner. My recollection of the evening was that it was perfect. I remember thinking about how this food was really fattening, though, and how it would make me fat if I kept it down. I didn't know or have the willpower to just not eat it. Over and over I tortured and berated myself about the effects this dinner would have on my body. I couldn't bear it. This dinner was no longer one meal; it was going to ruin my body and make me fat. I couldn't stand that food being inside me another moment. Looking back I can't imagine how I could have thrown up right there on the side of the road. It was like I had no couth. I told Matt to pull over, and I just stuck my hand down my throat. Rationalizing the act while engaging in it, I then jumped back in the truck to carry on with the night. We never discussed my vile act other than Matt saying, "I can't believe you just did that."

"I know," I responded, "but it just was making me feel so sick. I mean, my stomach was really nauseous."

Basically I don't know when I began this war with myself, but I know it caused me to fear myself. The rest is a blur—its beginning, its incentive. I heard Dr. Tant's question. I just didn't have the answer.

*Chelsea Browning Smith*
*September 7, 1992*

# A Precious Life

**Beverly Runyon**

ᗧ

I have never kept a journal or even a diary before. I know now that journaling is an accepted therapeutic tool, but I just never felt comfortable putting my daily feelings down in a tangible form. Maybe I had a problem with trust—what if someone read it someday? Maybe it was a way of staying in denial that my daughter might die.

To accurately recall how it all came about is difficult, because I am notorious for having a terrible memory. It is a family joke that I can never recall the event, conversation, or place the whole family is talking about. I now believe my poor memory has much to do with the problem I have of staying in the present moment. I have always been thinking about what I need to do next, what I ought to be doing, or should have done. My heart and mind are rarely totally present with me. I'm concerned about her or him, the what-ifs, the outcome. How could I remember taking in the cues, the clues, the hints, the hesitations, when my mind was not focused on the present? I am learning to slow down, to not be so hypervigilant. It is part of my recovery, part of my story, part of the journal I never took time to keep.

To now recall is also painful. Why would I want to remember what a few years ago kept me awake for hours as my mind swirled with thoughts of helping Chelsea and filled me

4

*with fear when I woke up exhausted in the morning? The first reason I am remembering and revealing the mistakes, the pain, and the truth now is that Chelsea asked me to. The second reason is that I believe in what she is doing to help others. If Chelsea is brave enough, caring enough, generous enough, honest enough to tell her story, then how could I not tell my part in it?*

*The first part of my life with Chelsea is not the best part, but it is a very close second. The first part is the first three years with Chelsea. When Chelsea was born, I was thirty-two years old, already the mother of two bright and beautiful children, nine-year-old daughter Ashley and almost-seven-year-old son John Holt. Chelsea was healthy and lovable, the happiest baby a person could hope for. She received tons of affection and attention from all of us and seemed to thrive on it.*

*The first year of her life was also one of the most difficult years of my life. That year it became apparent that my marriage of thirteen years was no longer something I could live with. Nor was it something I wanted my children to grow up with. My husband's extramarital affairs were a lifestyle I finally decided none of us deserved. We were separated shortly after Chelsea's first birthday, and the divorce was final when she was eighteen months old. My children were my source of strength and love during that painful time. Many a night I would go to Chelsea's crib when she was fast asleep. I would pick her up and cuddle her in a rocking chair. I might cry or softly sing a lullaby. She would never wake, yet her head on my shoulder and her cherub cheek on my cheek brought me more comfort than you can imagine. She was innately capable of nurturing and calming me then as well as now. I could sleep knowing that the divorce and single motherhood were worth the pain and fear.*

*Being a single mother of three was something I never*

*planned on or knew how I could accomplish. Supporting my three children was my most immediate concern. Securing a job was a result of being an active volunteer in the Junior League of Fort Worth. I had taken a leadership role through the Junior League in a project to prevent child abuse and neglect. The role resulted in the founding of the Parenting Guidance Center. I had served as the founding president of the board of directors for a time until Chelsea's birth, when I resigned from the presidency to have more time at home. However, I remained very active on the center's board of directors. Now I needed a paying job, and the center's executive director, Dorothy St. John, called me with one of the most appreciated offers I had ever received, a position on her staff.*

*Child care was never the major obstacle for me that it is for most single mothers. We are blessed with Mimi, my mother, who lives just several blocks away and who was always available to feed, carpool, entertain, discipline, spoil, and do all the wonderful things the best grandmother in the world would do. Ashley and John Holt had never had a baby-sitter thanks to Mimi's and Pampaw's (my father) open invitation and open hearts. Chelsea was just as welcomed, loved, and cherished in their home as she was in ours. I could go to work and financially support my children while my mother cared for them. Because we lived in the same neighborhood they could play with school and family friends. Mimi often had the children's friends and cousins over to play as well. My parents live on a dead-end street with little traffic, so when the children got bigger and more responsible they often played up and down the block with children of friends I had grown up with. Little did I know that this safe neighborhood play time would change everything.*

# Part One: 16–17 Years Old

*There is only one journey. Going inside yourself.*
—Rainer Maria Rilke

# *Fall 1992*

I could not get home fast enough. I had thought about that chocolate cake all day. I ran to the pantry and opened the freezer. You would have thought I was opening the gates of heaven. "I will just take this out and let it thaw; I just want to look at this chocolate dream." So I set it on the counter and watched. Then I decided that I needed to have some out and some in the freezer. I pressed the knife in a perfect horizontal position—awaiting the drop of a single morsel. Due to its below freezing temperature the cake held together like super glue. I reopened the gates—placing the magic wonder back where I would seize it another day. I sprinted the forty steps to the counter where the precut chocolate-on-chocolate sheet cake lay. This was a major "no way in hell" food; I would rather have someone chop off my tongue. I wondered what the cake would feel like if I microwaved it. Thirty-four seconds with a seventeen-second predefrost. Perfection was far too trite a word for the immaculate surrender of the melting icing flowing over the body of the cake onto the plate. And with that thought, I met my kiss of death. If someone had been listening and not known that this was a piece of cake, he would have thought I was making love to some long-lost lover. For the entire twenty minutes that damn chocolate cake became my world. I had to have it-not just one piece but several. Then I smashed the rest up and smeared it everywhere. I basically wanted to immerse myself in every morsel. I wanted us to become one. The affair ended all too soon. As my lover went out into the sewer, I felt like the most worthless person to have ever walked the earth. This was not the first time, and I am not ready for it to be my last. I just don't want to gain weight. And if I eat what I want I will.

I am getting better. I haven't thrown up in a week. But I started a new diet and workout with this fitness trainer, Steven. He is this old man but supposed to be great. Specializing in training pageant girls. No way in hell would I ever walk the runway, but to look like I have the body to is another thing. I couldn't believe these women asking Mom whether he was training me for my next pageant. I am so sure. Mom jumped on the opportunity to show me how I never see myself the way others do. I know they were thinking, "That poor girl, she doesn't have a prayer."

Anyway he changed my diet—grains and boiled chicken—and gave me a weight-lifting program in addition to my cardio. His goal is to tone and trim the fat. I was relived that he didn't want me to lose that much weight but to turn the fat into muscle. My goal is to find someone to tell me what to eat and help me stop feeling so guilty for everything I do eat. I don't know what to eat. I have myself so confused by all these rules. My rules are inconsistent in that I can have a whole yogurt one day and the next that would be too much (so I have to throw it up). I liked that he did not ask me to write down everything I eat. I hate how every nutritionist I go to does that. It is just this black and white reminder of how much I really eat. I pick and snack so much, having a bite here and there—those are impossible to record. I failed to mention my top priority is to lose weight. I don't know what perfect is anymore, all that matters is having a perfect body! Is that not sick? If I have a perfect body everyone will love me, I will be happy, and things will be so much easier. If I look right on the outside then eventually the inside will catch up. Where have you gone God? I need you please don't leave me.

ᏣᏂ-ᏣᎠ

What is happening? Things just get worse. Sometimes I hurt so much inside and I hate myself so much that I would rather die than feel as bad as I do. When I get this low, I can see nothing but death to make the pain just stop. I threatened to kill myself two times this break. But they weren't really threats, I wanted to. My plan was to take a whole lot of pills and just never wake up. I sprang this idea on Mom when she was taking me to the airport. I was going to meet Dad in Charleston for Christmas. I did not want to go. I told her that this was it. If I had to go I would kill myself. I was crying—so was she. I don't know what she was thinking or feeling. All I knew was my own desperate need to escape from myself and from the world I had come to know. I am so fucked up. As I walked down the gate she looked at me as though she truly feared never seeing me again. The crazy part is that of all the people on earth, she was the one I wanted to hurt least and the one I never wanted to leave.

I called her from the airport where I had a layover. I reassured her that I would be fine and apologized. She hates me and probably wishes I had done it. I don't know what brought all these intense feelings on, but I felt like I had the world on my shoulders and that there was no one on this planet worse than me or more screwed up. I just don't know what to do with anything. I felt like it was the only way I could get them to take me seriously and to know that I was so miserable. I don't know what to do. I just want this to all stop. I hate my life and how depressed I am. I really don't think it will ever get better, and I don't know whether I want to wait around to see. What would they think if I did kill myself? I wonder if they would miss me or if they would blame themselves? They would be sad for a while, but they would all go on. I would be remembered as that wasted life. This just sucks. Now I need to make everything be okay when I see my dad. I don't want to get him into all this. He doesn't have a clue what hell it is to live with me. He and Jude would probably make light of the whole thing. This is really serious to me.

☙❧

I made it to Charleston and did not throw up for three weeks—but then I blew it. Being with all these strangers or extended family and my dad and stepmother did something to me. Dad has some interesting relatives and we had fun, but I couldn't forget the things I had done at the airport—the big mess I stirred up back home. Mom just sounded terrified on the phone and I feel horrible that I made her hurt so much. Looking back on Christmas '92, it was a disaster thanks to me. I am a little spoiled brat. Mom tries so hard and no matter what she does, how she says it, or how she does it, I still am pathetic. She can't make it better for me. I almost wish she would tell me to "Fuck off" and "if I want to live this way go right ahead." She runs around trying to make everything go smoothly and make it a perfect Christmas for twenty-something people. It is impossible. I wish she would give it a rest. It's hard not to be a little annoyed by someone trying so hard. Of course I just sink my feet further into my bad mood and want to be skinny all the more. The thinner I get the louder I scream "Fuck you, I am doing this my way and you can't make me change."

# Spring 1993

Dad called and said that he wants to take John Holt and me to Rome for spring break with Jude. That would be pretty cool if he follows through.

Dr. Tant and I have been talking about my parents the past few sessions. They have never really said why they got a divorce except that things didn't work out between them and that they weren't happy. I have always had this gut feeling that there was more of a story there, even the possibility of my dad having had an affair. Dr. Tant and I talked about ways I would bring up the question. And so I did.

Mom and I had just pulled into the garage. We had been shopping for most of the day. I just kept that thinking for as long as I could remember I had wanted to know the truth about the divorce. I finally gutted up and said, "Mom did Dad have an affair?" There was a long silence. "Yes, but I never wanted to tell you. I didn't want you to hold it against your father, and I never thought it was something you needed to know." I was shocked. I could not believe that he could cheat on Mom. Even though I had always thought that's what had happened, having my assumption confirmed created a whole new side of my dad—one that I almost wish I had never come to know. The act of cheating is horrible enough, but the repercussions are hard to excuse. I can't help but think that by com-

14

mitting those acts he prohibited us from living together. In a way it was like he cheated on all of us. I really don't care to hear any excuses. He screwed up and lost so much, I almost feel sorry for him. What a fool to give up so much for sex.

I feel so incredibly guilty. I was baby-sitting my niece this afternoon and I don't know why but I got this dumb idea to take ipecac, which makes you throw up. I drank a lot of it. I got really sick and of course called Mom. I know it was all about attention. They were all really pissed. How self-centered and dumb of me. Mom just let me lie there by the toilet all night and throw up. I don't know why I wanted her attention so badly. I really want them to know that I am hurting and am capable of doing whatever it is that I am trying to accomplish. I guess that I am successful in my disease, as sick as that sounds. I wanted her to care for me and nurture me—I wanted her to love me. I wanted her to tell me it would all go away and I would be okay. She seems so troubled by me and I want to know she still cares. I won't take that stuff anymore.

∞∞

What do they think I do after dinner? When I get up from the table I tiptoe out of the kitchen and hope they don't ask where I am going. Are they fools for not knowing? The fact that they are so trusting or oblivious makes my secret all the worse. It is such a painful secret, but I always know I will feel better after I get it all out. I have no right to have that much dinner.

I don't care what I do—I can't stop throwing up. I hate myself so much for doing it. I try so hard not to. I am falling apart. I am so fat, I am so disgusting. I deserve where I am putting my head. I am screwing up my body beyond repair. My throat and lungs are killing me. Why am I still doing this? I hardly eat, and I feel so guilty for eating even one meal. When I start bingeing I am not hungry and I don't think about the act—I just stuff and stuff. My system is used to it. It doesn't even digest the food for a long time. If I get fat, my life and purpose are over. Why does this lying thought control my life? God help me, PLEASE! I am begging you. I wish my mom could comfort me. I don't know how to love myself or really remember what there is to love about me. I don't want her to go on that trip. My eating will only get worse. Every time I hear someone coming in the kitchen I throw away whatever I am eating because the person might think that I shouldn't be eating. I don't want them to think about how much I eat and I don't want them to comment on what I am eating. I try my hardest to read their minds, to discern what they think when they see me in the kitchen snacking.

∞∞

Dad called and said that we are going to Rome for spring break. John Holt, Jude, Dad, and I will go for fifteen days. I know they will catch me if I throw up. I know I can't while I am there. They will watch me like crazy.

∞∞

Now this is strange. It has been forever since I last wrote. Well to catch you up, I made a big decision the day before I went to Rome that I was not going to throw up anymore. Well, I also had some help because my dad, Jude, and John Holt (whom I love more than anything) would be watching me like hawks. I don't know how and can't explain it, but I just made up my mind that throwing up is bad and I want to stop. Besides it wouldn't be that hard I thought because, "I don't have a real serious problem." There were times when I thought I would explode, but I did not want to get into it with them. Little did I know at first that I had a plan number two. Since I was not going to throw up, I would just not eat. I am not and was not ready to give this thing up. Besides, my dad doesn't have a clue what living with me is like—especially with an eating disorder. All he gets are the secondhand stories. This trip would be a crash course in a day in hell, Chelsea's life. He definitely got a sense of the extreme effort I devote to nurturing this disease. I would order a plain salad and put vinegar on the plain lettuce. They tried everything. They even learned in Italian how to say no oil or butter. I still would laugh inside because no matter what they did to bring my meal up to "healthy" standards I was not going to eat it. They would find something I would eat at one meal, and based on the morsel I let touch my lips at the previous one, search for the next restaurant. I basically stopped eating. It scared me how much my actions affected my family. I think they are starting to see what a hell I live in and how miserable I am. It was John Holt's first day-to-day encounter with my problem and he hated it. I feel bad because in some ways I wanted the trip to be great, but I also wanted to receive attention and to feel that they cared about me. But most of all I wanted them to let me eat as I wanted to. If anything ruined the trip it was my grave attempt to fill my self-centered need.

∞∞

My mom and Bill just left for a trip, and I am going to move in with Elizabeth and her parents. Mom and Bill have made it perfectly clear that I am a little bitch who causes them only stress and trouble. I am rude to Bill. I hate that I am not sweet to him, but I really resent that he is always lecturing me about something, looking for what I do wrong, and never noticing my desire to do everything just right. All he talks to me about is food, food, and fat. It drives me nuts. I hate it, so I make little bitchy remarks to try and defuse some of my anger. Well it is not working. I guess I am still pissed over what he said to me in the kitchen before I left for Rome. I had just come in from working out and he had just come in the door from work. "Hey Bill. How was work?"

"Oh it was a hard day. I had a ton of patients." I continued making my salad. He came over next to me to wash his hands at the sink. The uncomfortable silence was quickly filled. "Chelsea, you look great. You have trimmed down and look really great."

"Thanks, Bill." That compliment was uncomfortable enough. I wish he had stopped there. He went on.

"You know I was starting to get worried about you. I mean you were really putting on the weight. I am so relieved you have gotten it under control. I wasn't sure you would."

I smiled and gave a slight chuckle. As always I swallowed my real feelings. I knew this painful and twisted compliment would be replayed continually in my mind, and be rehearsed countless times a day. For me at that moment, Bill represented every unspeaking male in the world. He was just the only one who had the nerve to come out and say how fat and disgusting I had become. How could I walk the earth and have the nerve to hold my head high when in reality all these people had been thinking or saying, "Man she looks like shit," "She has let herself go," or "She has put on the pounds"? From that day forth I vowed to never, ever let anyone think again that I had "put on the pounds" or that I had let myself become this fat, worthless, piece of trash.

As for Mom, she has had it with me. She is just exhausted by the sight of me. It is obvious I am no longer a joy. It's as though she is counting down the days until we are apart. She doesn't even like showing me affection anymore. She talks about clothes with me and gives me compliments like a routine overly rehearsed, attempting to understand where her futile efforts to instill strong self-esteem went sour. I feel sorry for her as she continues to try to make something get through.

She buys me things all the time, thinking the clothes will make me happy, or maybe that is how she tells me she cares. It used to be different. All I want is for her to spend time with me, loving me and talking with me. Maybe that's bad that I love her so and that I need my mom so much, but right now that is the way it is. She told me not to read her mind, but I told her that I have to sometimes because she never expresses her feelings. It is not about reading her mind anymore. It is crying out of her eyes and plastered across her body that her last child is a nightmare to live with and that she is a failure. All I want when I get mad at my mom is a reaction from her, but that is something that she will not do. She never has lost her temper or shown how much something makes her mad or expressed much of any negative feeling. She is always very controlled. I just wish she would scream at me. I deserve it. I am such a disappointment. I had so many things I was doing right. I thought my life looked so promising and that I would be the one that would make her eyes sparkle with joy. I don't know what I am now, and I don't know what I need to be now. But I know this is killing her.

⌒⌒⌒

When I talked to Mom on the phone we quickly fell into our familiar roles. She and I both pretended that nothing had happened, like we had never gotten into a fight before she left for New York. I don't get how can she just pretend like everything is okay.

Alicia told me that everyone asks her whether I am anorexic. Alicia has been one of my best friends since we were little kids and she really tries to not step on my toes, so we never talk about it. When she tells me stuff like that I just laugh and say how crazy they all are, which I really do believe. People are making way too big of a deal out of this. I am glad that she defends me and is not on anyone's side because people have really started gossiping about my weight loss. I really don't talk about it with any of my friends. I can tell they watch me, but the only time they ever say stuff is when other people are bugging them, wondering whether I am okay. No one has just come out and said I want to help you. All I know of are the secondhand conversations that occasionally I am retold. I wonder whether it scares them or whether they even think about it. I don't want them to worry or for it to turn them away. I really don't think it should freak them out. I can stop whenever, and I really am in control of this. They don't need to worry. I just feel so much better about myself. I hate how mothers are always making comments to me about how "emaciated" I am, as if I were some kind of freak. No wonder I don't want to go out of my house. I would be better in a freakshow the way people react to how different I look. Their comments don't help. I wish they would just say "I love you" or "I care about you" and not just look at the outside. The inside is what hurts. I don't blame them for not understanding. They try to relate to the symptoms, which don't make complete sense even to me. They should be left at that, mere symptoms. I believe the truth lies at the symptoms' roots. Trying to understand their source might be a great investment, but this deeper understanding is far more tangible. It must hurt pretty bad for me to do all this. People just seem to look at me so sadly—almost as though I am in decay. Don't they realize they only make things worse? I am finally getting pleased with my body. I like that I can feel my hip bones and that my thighs don't touch at all. I like that my arms are small enough for my hand to barely close around them. All my clothes are very loose, even the ones I bought just a few weeks ago. It scares me that I know I am thinner, but I don't see it like they do. I just want to lose a little more. It's weird that I want some people to think I have a problem and to know how hard I try, but then when they notice I wish they would leave me alone. Others I pray won't notice.

Sometimes I feel like it is revenge, because I think things like, "I'll show you," maybe toward Mom and Dad. Part of me wants to do this to my mom. I am angry with her because she needs so much to please—she is weak. She lets my dad get away with rarely paying child support or paying for school. She never tells Bill what she wants but expects him to know, or she does what he wants. The frustrating part is that she is an amazing woman and offers so much when she does speak her mind. I just hate it because I can read her like a book, and I know her sweet voice and smile do not truthfully reflect what she is feeling all the time. She deserves so much more and in some sense prohibits herself from going out and doing or getting what she wants. Gosh, why is this making me cry? I don't want to let anyone dictate my needs or give them so much power over me that it ultimately stifles my dreams. Another part makes me sad because I hate how I create the exhausted look on her face and in her body. It kills me to see her like that.

I usually don't think about what is driving me. It is more automatic, almost instinctive, so the motive may change most of the time. I really think I just want to be thin, but a lot of people want to be thin and don't go to the extreme I do. I am relieved that I have not thrown up, and it feels good.

Sometimes I want there to be a problem so I will know I am doing my job well. I put so much energy into my body and worrying about what goes into it. But maybe in some weird way I have chosen to destroy my body in hopes that "they" will see that I am dying inside. I guess I feel like I can't just say it. I've become determined to show them what my insides feel like. I don't think I will ever understand the constant war going on inside my head. I think my breathing problem is sort of neat, whether it has anything to do with my eating deal. I get out of breath walking up stairs and my heart feels really strange—almost heavy. When I went to the doctor she said it was asthma, but I have never had anything like this until two months ago. She freaked out when she saw how low my pulse and heart rate were. Then she started in—thinking that she was going to introduce the idea that I could have an eating disorder. I just zoned out.

She tried to talk to me about eating disorders. You know, the usual. "Anorexia nervosa is a extreme weight-loss condition, typically where a woman or girl drops at least fifteen percent of her body weight." I tuned in just enough to nod my head at the appropriate time. I had heard the same spiel every time the word eating disorder was spoken. I couldn't help but wonder whether she was really naive or overly optimistic about the effect my level of knowledge on the subject matter could have. Statistics were not going to change anything. I lived this. I didn't need to hear the numbers and be convinced how serious this disease was. Maybe I should have described some of my meals in order to quiet her redundancy. Like how thinly I slice my bread or how I measure the single teaspoon of milk for my coffee—anymore I throw out. I eat healthy stuff, mostly vegetables and frozen yogurt. I eat a lot of tomatoes and broccoli. It sounds bad, but it is good. I don't know when I'll be satisfied with my efforts or whether I will ever believe that I truly fit this textbook description of an anorexic.

I always dreamed of being five feet eight inches and 115 pounds, and now I am far below but still not satisfied. I always imagined myself being skinny, like the girls on a runway or in a magazine. Then I would be skinny enough. I mean, that is the way we all aspire to be. It is the ideal. I wish I could accurately see myself as other people do. It is exhausting trying to be what I think I should be—trying to maintain those high ideals and standards.

ꝏꝏ

You know, when people comment about my weight I feel like they are intruding on my privacy, like they are watching me.

It is weird how Lauren and I are far apart when we used to be so close. I guess it is sort of like the rest of my friends. I don't do that much with any of them anymore. I just don't like to. Brad told me that Lauren feels like I am controlling and manipulative. It broke my heart. I would never want to hurt her. She has been my best friend since birth.

I think about who I write to in my journal. It seems to change, but I guess mostly I write to God. Sometimes I hope that my mom finds it when I die. I need to be stronger than that and not let people control my feelings so much or be so damn dependent. Since my mom has been out of town it has been good. I have had to deal with things on my own. I have to believe that things happen for a reason and that God will help me out of this pain.

ꝏꝏ

What happened to my dream of being a lawyer in the most prestigious law firm in America? Since the sixth grade I've always wanted to go to Vanderbilt Law School and become a hotshot female lawyer. I loved the idea of being powerful, independently successful and following in my father's footsteps. I can't say when my dream began to change—now I struggle to recall the person who believed in myself enough to fulfill that dream. I would really like to be a lawyer, maybe go into politics. It's sad how my biggest dream has faded to a mere reflection. It scares me how things are becoming a reality so fast. No longer do I believe in my ability to fulfill my strongest aspirations, much less my desire for a fulfilling life. I just want things to be right. I don't want to be dependent on anyone, especially some man.

I want to go to heaven so badly. I think it will be great. I can't do this life right. No matter what I do my choices are never good enough. I don't want to look back and regret my life and say, "What a screw up." I need to pass time right now because the longer I do, the longer before I eat. I love those times when I can eat one bite without guilt—usually when I am in physical pain (so, so hungry) or really sick. I then feel I deserve to eat. You know, I think I try to be really involved in school partly so that I can tell Mom, because when I tell her I can see how happy it all makes her. I don't have a life. I want to hide from myself the reality of how shallow my world has become. If I think about it for too long I really start to beat myself up. My world and my perspective have not always been so bleak, so small or debilitating. Sometimes I wonder what "I" really enjoy doing. I have really begun to realize that all the food in the world is not going to change my feelings or problems and that it is going to take time for me to love myself—loving the little girl I used to be. I love to remember my perception of myself and the innocent way I viewed the world. I am sad that the joy I had as a child is a memory, no longer a reality. I must not forget but recall what I once had and what I believe still exists. I will get through this and win. I know I have it in me.

ꙮ

I am half through one of the most incredible experiences I've ever had. I am taking a course in self-defense called Model Mugging. It is unbelievable. We did some amazing stuff. I broke a board with my foot today, using the hammer kick.

What really freaked me out was practicing being assaulted lying down. It was as if the mugger was Michael on top of me. I really got nauseated. I could not stop the tears. I was terrified and I just wanted to knock the shit out of him so he would get off of me. I was so afraid to cry in front of the class. I felt like they would think I was exaggerating or being overly dramatic. Even though they didn't know what had happened with Michael, they reassured me that my tears were okay. Ultimately I kicked the mugger's ass.

Tomorrow the mugger will completely reenact the afternoon with Michael. I cannot wait to knock the shit out of Michael. Knowing that I am learning to defend myself and, most of all, protect against what I could not at the age of four is the best feeling. It is an eerie feeling to look in the mirror and see the darkness in my eyes. I know this darkness was never meant to be part of me. That day left a nasty feeling. It's a feeling that makes you think a piece of you is already dead. I have always wondered whether I will ever see a way to bring it back. It was an afternoon that, for me, has never ended. I'll die kicking and screaming before I ever let someone take my innocence away again (if it's something that can be stolen twice).

One of the girls in the class asked me if I was anorexic. How do people tell? The instructor/mugger was very impressed with my strength "considering how small and thin" I am. I don't like talking to the group about my feelings. I don't know what to say. I told them how I hate when women are verbally harassed by men. I can't stand them staring, like workmen and guys in cars or in school walking down the halls; so of course the instructor thrives on that when he pretends to be the mugger. He will say everything and anything to really get me riled up when we are practicing. Mom, Mimi, and Dr. Tant came to the graduation. They were pretty shocked. I don't think they knew what to expect. I have a videotape and I can't wait to show Lauren. She will crack up.

☙❧

My mom is in Aspen and I miss her so much. It bothers me that I can't go on like any other sixteen-year-old would if her parents were gone and be happy inside. Instead I get really sad and lonely. Sometimes I have to get really mad at her before she goes. It makes her leaving easier. The harder she tries to make me happy the angrier I get. I don't think I can ever overcome this deep attachment. It is so strong and solid. I feel so empty inside and it didn't help to be rude to her. It only made me feel guilty. I wish I could just cry, but it is so hard. Tomorrow is a day that I have been dreading like the plague—cheerleading practice starts. I feel so alone, disliked, and isolated. I am scared of how all these girls will act around me. I know that I look different and that my weight has really dropped. People are always shocked when they have not seen me for awhile. They get really freaked out. I hate that! The girls think I am some freak and look at me like I am crazy. All my relationships with them have become very superficial and shallow. I guess they don't know what to say to me. That is so dumb. I am still the same person.

⚬⚬⚬

I feel like shit today. I just got back from Fort Lauderdale after a vacation with my mom and some of our family friends. I have gained three and a half pounds. I can't forgive myself. I am so scared I am going to get huge or keep gaining weight. I have got to stop it. This is driving me nuts. I am completely obsessing about this. The dumb thing on my part is that I wanted to get up to 110 because I thought the extra weight would make people shut up! The pictures from cheerleading camp scared me. I look so thin and my nose sticks out. My face looked hard and gaunt and my eyes dark. But I know one thing—gaining three pounds to make everyone else happy has made me feel like shit. I will shed them A.S.A.P. if it kills me. These people are being way too extreme to call me anorexic. I am not that good, and I am not that thin. I can tell that I am skinnier, but that is mostly because I wear a size one and not the size six I did less than a year ago. A size one is small, but I don't really look that small and I am not anorexic.

❧

I have set myself up to fail. My standard is to be as perfectly thin as a model. I won't love myself until I get there. They are the way to look. Every guy drools over them; every woman envies them. They are on every magazine cover—they must do something right. I feel like it would be worthwhile, right now, to be this strict with my thinking and regimen. I have put all these pictures of Kate Moss on the inside of my closet and on my mirror in my bathroom. I suck, I am ugly, and I don't understand how anyone could give me a compliment. They must give compliments because it is polite. I feel so disgusting with these rolls of fat hanging on my body.

❧

God, things in my life are so strange right now. I wonder each day whether I will be lucky enough to get through without being confronted with my thinness. People constantly talk about it. I get so tired of hearing how "emaciated" I supposedly am. Trying to create new alibis is getting old. I wish I would be left alone. I want to strangle someone every time I hear the key phrase "you are so skinny." I think, or at least they say, that my drastic weight change is what freaks people out. They don't know what to think.

I always look forward to tomorrow or some future event that will make me happy. I look forward to the next day because it is a fresh start to eat just right. But the weird thing is that it's never right. I cook a lot, but I never eat what I cook. I chew up the food, cram as much in my mouth as I can, and then spit it out in the sink. I will do this over and over. At least I am not throwing up. Today I ate some chocolate pudding and rice. I hate it when I do eat because I think about it all day, pinching the fat on my stomach to increase the guilt or maybe to remind myself that I am not good enough. I am scared to death that I will go over 110. I am much more comfortable with 107. You know, I really don't see myself as skinny as everyone says. I actually laugh at all the people getting involved because I don't see it as a problem like everyone else does. Sure I obsess about what I eat and I do get full. I think I am close to having an eating disorder, but anorexia? No. I am not nearly that thin. I love being a size two or one. It is just perfect. The biggest mistake I have made is trying to gain weight for other people. I have ripped myself up inside over three pounds. I do want to get better. I especially want to live in the present and not feel guilt about the past. Tomorrow I want more than anything to be perfectly content with right now!

I fear my senior year because it is such a moment of truth. Where will I go to school? I want so badly to go to Vanderbilt if they will take me. See? My happiness and drive are all based on things I have no control over.

∞∞

Dear God, please help ease my anxieties. I am so afraid to go to school. I am terrified people won't like me if I am skinny. I don't want to lose my place. I don't want to be an outcast. I just want to hide. Help them see it is the same person under this skin. I love you with all my heart.

∞∞

I started thinking about what my friends and I do when we go out at night. I was confused many times and not sure what to feel. I get frustrated because I don't like going to bars. We can't all get in and our efforts usually result in embarrassment. Then we start driving around from one place to another or just sit and drink at someone's house. It gets really old. That is pretty much what my friends do. The rest have boyfriends and stay home and rent movies. I really don't like to put all that crap in my body or smell all the smoke. I really love to go to dinner with my parents or maybe a movie. I like it when I have a low-key night with my friends, but it doesn't happen often. The truth is that I don't like to go out. I don't like to leave my house. I want to be around food and I don't want to be put in a situation that might make me uncomfortable, like guys going on and on about how skinny I am. When I am away from my house I am terrified. Fear controls all my thoughts. What if I eat or drink too much and I gain too much weight? What if I am not able to get up and work out the next day like I need to? When I am away from food I think about it and miss it as though it were a person, and I long to reside in the refuge of our relationship. I am in pain—even anguish—when I am away.

# Fall 1993

I am crying right now! Right now! I usually never cry. I was starting to believe it wasn't possible anymore. I am so weighed down by this bag of shit I have been carrying around that I could die. I get so overwhelmed and obsessed with the things I should be doing or saying. When I get bored I go crazy. I get like this. I think all the time, but when I am still, I have to feel. I am so confused inside. I don't want my birthday to come. I am dreading it. I know no matter what happens it won't be perfect enough. I won't do it right. I swear if I were given the Hope diamond I would not be happy. Not because I wouldn't love it or would be ungrateful but because I know I don't deserve anything. It's not that I am spoiled. I really would rather get nothing. I am not surprised I always get let down by gifts, because I have this weird belief that a present shows how much a person values you.

I don't want any big deal made out of this stupid day. I can't be myself on my birthday. I have to be or act a way I don't feel. I feel like my birthday is my day and everything should be "perfectly" my way. But I don't even know what that is, so how could I expect someone else to know? I would rather it be forgotten. I remember how birthdays growing up were the best. They could make everything joyous for the whole month before and the month to follow. I know that this birthday—my seventeenth—won't take away what I have done or what I am. Nor will it bring anyone joy. All I want to have is one healthy living moment. I would give anything to have it for five minutes.

I hate seeing the sadness I bring to my mom's face when she tries so hard to make me happy and then realizes she can't. I hate being her last child. I can't be the girl I think she would be proud to claim. I feel so guilty that I am fucking up, ruining her last experiences of bringing up a child. I want to be perfect for her, to make her happy and fulfilled by her wonderful child. I know that sounds pathetic, but I really believe that this is my rightful duty—my role in the family. My brother and sister are different from me, and I need to be this way. I hate that I am failing.

ॐ

Dr. Tant told me the coolest thing today: "Shame is the internal fear of being exposed. All perfection comes from shame."

I ripped myself apart in aerobics. I had so much anger, energy, that I wanted to literally rip my body apart and work it until I dropped. I was going crazy. I have been eating more but have not been feeling guilty as I usually do. So for that I am going to punish myself tomorrow. I won't eat hardly a thing and I'm going to work out.

How can I hang pictures of Kate Moss all over my bathroom as a person to strive to be? I could never do it that well. I want to hide my face. I am ashamed. I don't want people to see how ugly it really is. I try to cover the ugly, bad parts. I guess if you sum it up I have lost my power and control. If I don't believe in myself then why should anyone else? I hate that. I am so sick of everything being reduced to that. People try to simplify my eating thing into a control issue. Come on! It cannot be that simple. I've decided I don't want people to look at me. I am so ashamed I am not better.

I lost this weight and I love the way my body looks and feels. It is a great rush being a size two or zero. I live for it. So for a couple of days I have been easing the guilt. I try to gain and lose at the same time, as crazy as that is. If I can stay this way or maybe a little smaller, not much, then I would be happier with myself. I look thin in those pictures, but anything is better than the pig I was, with the excess crap I had all over my body. When I do eat more spontaneously or eat as I please, thoughts of throwing up come to mind. It scares the shit out of me because sometimes I just want to stuff the whole bowl of rice down my throat or to make something sweet, eat the batter, and just make it all come out. I love to just immerse myself in it, get it all over my face. I just can't get enough. Will I ever find a balance? I don't feel like I deserve anything or that I am worth anything. I pick my skin constantly. I am so angry at myself for not being enough or good enough. How can I feel good about myself when my greatest urge is to put my head in a toilet?

I have really started believing that I am just ugly. I look weird and all out of proportion. What am I even suppose to look like? What is a normal weight? How do I eat normally? I want to look pretty, so maybe I need to gain a little weight. But then the other part of me loves the way my body feels. I love to touch my thighs and feel my butt bones and my hip bones. I love my bones showing across my chest and the bones on my shoulders. There is no extra fluff that excites me. I love being the size I am. Bigger seems worthless, bad. I want more than anything to love, value, and do the most with the way I am and stop comparing myself to others, picking myself apart. I can stand almost forever in a trance in front of the mirror. Staring so long and hard at one minute section of my leg, turning just so to prove that my legs are gross, almost to confirm my repetitive thoughts that they are getting larger before my eyes.

I am not going to take these stupid birth control pills much longer because I have been trying my ass off to lose weight and I'm not. But I will! I had to go to the gynecologist because I stopped having a period a while back. She told me how it is so important for my body to get the proper amount of estrogen and that I needed to take birth control pills to get my system on track. Despite the fact that she promises there are not any side effects, I don't believe her. I know that is why I feel so fat. I want to be thin and I'll be damned if I get fat and start having a period again. I am dying to figure out a new way to lose weight. Screw all these people who say I am too skinny. I love it. Besides most of my friends are on my side supporting my "recovery"—the recovery that I am desperately fighting. I am not about to not give up any of my ways. I would rather die than get all gross and fat. I love convincing people that I don't want to be this way and I want to give all this up. The reason I like to convince people is that they leave me alone and will not talk to me about it. I get tired of just hearing about how thin I am. I can't believe that they really will believe me when I tell them how hard I am trying and how much I want to get better. I know it's not right to lie to all of them, but what else can I say? If I told them the truth there's no telling what would happen. I am not ready to give in or up, but I don't want them to alienate me because they think I am weird. If better equals fat I want no part of it. Damn I am screwed up.

I don't know how to talk to God anymore. I need to talk to someone about my isolation from him. Does God still love me? Does he really exist? I don't hear him like I used to. Was I just imaging the whole thing?

I am so proud! I can't believe the scale today. I weigh 103. That is simply amazing. I am determined to handle this in a healthy way. I mean I need to ease up on myself and not try to lose more weight; 103, this is good. I know I have not written in forever. I have so much to tell. I did great while my parents were in Europe. Dad came in for homecoming. It was wonderful. But the best surprise of all was Bret, my homecoming date. The date was sort of set up. I had seen him around school and always thought he was so hot. Then when I heard he broke up with his girlfriend, a little networking to get a date with him seemed only appropriate. I can't remember the last time I have ever gone out with someone so sweet. We had such a blast together. I really like hanging out with him. I get excited to see him when I go to school. I have felt great lately! I feel healthy and happy. God really has answered my prayers. I have thought about my feelings and how needy I am, but it is so hard for me to admit that I need other people, as well as their love.

∽∾

It is amazing, it is like no time has passed. For the past four days I have been throwing up for whatever reason or excuse I could think of. It has been since March that I was consecutively throwing up. What is going on? I mean I am sitting yakking on the phone and the next thing I know I am overeating (more than I plan), then my head is in the toilet until my body begins to dry heave. I don't want to face tomorrow. I want to hide. When I chose to stop throwing up, my solution to the problem was to stop eating. I became disgusted by the whole idea of throwing up. Now it seems like old times. My hardest time tends to be at night. I am scared to death to turn this over to God. But God, I have had it. I don't want to write, go to aerobics, go to school, fill out college applications, or take any damn birth control pills. I can hardly even talk to you anymore, God. I don't know how to begin to live anymore. I don't know this person I have become. In just two years I have become a stranger to myself. I am consumed by my thoughts, living in this hell my mind has created. I never wanted it to be this way. Being this way has never made me happy. The crazy part is, I keep on because I am afraid. I am just terrified, maybe of failing everyone, not fulfilling my responsibilities, not making things right, or not doing anything right. I am deathly afraid of my humanity—the reality that I won't ever do it right. I fear my inability to fulfill what I believe is my role. What is going on?

⌒⌒⌒

I think about cooking all the time and immersing myself in food. When I am in school, all I can think about is food. I eat so many pieces of gum, and I freak out over the eight to ten calories in each piece. And I forgot about my eating a blow pop, fifty calories. That is probably what has kept my weight on.

Get this. While I was cooking yesterday I stabbed my hand with a knife trying to get this bottle open. The knife was just sticking out of my hand. I couldn't feel anything. I knew I had to get it out. I think I was in shock. The skin hung on the serrated edge. As I pulled its tip out, blood poured. The next thing I remembered was hearing my body hit the floor. Mom got me up and tied my hand tight until we got to the doctor. The shot hurt like hell. Right between my fingers and thumb. I couldn't watch him pull the string in and out. It hurt like hell to get stitches. I am always cutting myself. I don't mean to, but when I cut the thin, thin, thin slices of bread or whatever I am cooking it is hard not to.

I hate that I don't have the same lunch period as my friends anymore. They have second lunch period and I have first. Not that I would go with them. They would be staring at my food and I would feel so paranoid. It is just easier to eat alone. My lunch is becoming rather routine. The people at the frozen yogurt shop know me by name. I love to get the large size but it takes me so long to make up my mind on the flavor.

I think it really irritates them. If someone comes with me to lunch I take a few bites in front of them and then go to the bathroom and throw the rest out. If I am alone I will just dump the rest in the trash. I get so hungry and worn out, but I am still sticking to my new routine of aerobics twice a day. I go to the 6:00 A.M. and then one of the afternoon classes. I just really have to psych myself up to do it sometimes. I am obsessed with this woman in my aerobics class who is absolutely beautiful. She is really anorexic, but I swear she has to have been a model. I would give anything to follow her around for just one day and see how she does it. What she does to make herself so successful at starving and looking great. I bet she is so good. When she is not in class I like to get in her spot. You can see in her eyes how focused she is—she doesn't even notice anyone else in the room. Her determination is amazing. She works so hard and has so much energy. She stares in the mirror and is just incredible. I think I see her differently than other people might. When I told Lauren how awesome I thought she was Lauren freaked out that I liked the way she looked. But I don't care. If I could be like her I would be awesome. I bet she weighs no more than ninety pounds and has to be at least five-foot ten. I cannot do anything about being five eight, but I can lose some more weight.

I am so addicted to food I always have to have something in my mouth, especially sweet things. I always stay busy. I am so disgusting. All that matters is my losing five more pounds, even if it kills me.

☙ ❧

Tonight I realized the truth about myself, even though the truth is not pretty. Now that I know it exists I can deal with it. As I was getting ready for this father/daughter dance, I realized how badly I wanted to look good but how much I couldn't stand the way I actually looked. I could feel this rage inside me grow, and as I began to think about my feelings of inadequacy, I began to realize how empty I have been on the inside. I don't really care, feel, or think about much. I feel so guilty. Once I got to the party I found myself wondering if these girls hated themselves as much as I hate myself. Do they beat themselves up the way I do myself every day? Am I normal? I almost hoped that I wasn't the freak I felt I was. That I wasn't alone with these thoughts that control my world and have changed the course of any life I had once dreamed I would live. I know deep down that not many people would choose to get up every day if they woke to the same voice I do. Believe me, it is not a privileged life. Does anyone else tell herself how worthless she is? That if she takes a bite of that lettuce with oily dressing she will get fat? That even if she does eat she is worthless and stupid and can't accomplish anything? My mind sorts through ultimatums. These threats are futile attempts to hang on to the familiarity and comfort of the hell I have created. I simply cannot give in to my desire to eat. I don't know. I am the most evil person on the inside, so incredibly hateful. I feel like I am in the same range as a serial rapist, except that I rape myself of any hope of a different life, one lived without internal hate.

⌬

I hate food, I am so fucking addicted to it! I swear it's like I can't come home once and get out of the kitchen without something to eat. It is as if the kitchen has a personality—not a human personality—but one of an evil demon. This monster is so full of life for me that it is everything. It is my joy, my pain, and my god. I really believe that it is alive. In some way I guess it has to be. I feel so passionate about everything that happens in there. It really is my life support, and it knows all my secrets, even the ones I dare not even tell myself. I make myself full not just of food but of feelings that are not even mine. Sometimes I can't even breathe so I suffer or throw up. I really don't do well when I talk on the phone in the kitchen because I will eat every bite without thinking about the repercussions, then feel really guilty. I suck so bad; I have been snacking even when I am not hungry. Nothing pisses me off more than when I am eating and someone interrupts me or the phone rings. When someone comes in the kitchen and looks at me, especially Mom, it's like it is all over her face how screwed up I am and how I really have no need to be eating. I try to stop but I can't. I don't want to go to bed. I know if I wake up the next day it will be worse than the day I just left. I dread school, the fear of the unexpected. I also fear hearing people say how sick I am and knowing that I will not eat right tomorrow. I know I will eat too much—and always the wrong stuff.

I can't control this addiction. It scares me. Please help! I do it when I am happy, too. I can't beat this on my own. I can't believe I was put here on earth to be an eating disorder and spend the rest of my life in a toilet or smashing food down the sink. I want so much to have a life some day with a husband and children. I am so scared that I may not be able to if I keep this up. I am terrified that I may never believe I deserve more than I now have.

# Winter 1994

My brand new journal with the new year. I am going to work really hard at writing as close to every day as possible. I am choosing for my new year's resolution to not throw up, to find God, and to deal with things in a healthy way. I still weigh 108 and would love to weigh less, but I don't feel like starving right now. I am scared. I don't want to fail.

I plan on talking to Dr. Tant about how I feel like such a bad and dirty kid. I figure I feel this way because of Michael. I am so ashamed. When I look at four-year-old little girls, it amazes me that anyone could ever touch them in an unloving way. How could someone rip into their gentle hearts? It is crazy for me to think even for a second that it was my fault. Something has happened to make me believe that I could have had control over that sixteen-year-old man, that I could have somehow made that afternoon turnout different. Now my body tells me it was my fault. I'll never know to what degree my thoughts are a byproduct of the event or to what extent it shaped the person I have become. I wish I knew how much or in what way he colored my thoughts and inhibitions. I do know a part of me was left in his room that afternoon. Still I see it all through the same little-girl eyes. So it's not hard to believe my demon still lives.

I feel so much love and hope when I see little children. Nothing makes me more happy. The thought of anyone stealing and trampling their innocence breaks my heart. It has broken my heart. I wish someone would have hurt him or had really gotten mad about the whole deal. Not a day since that afternoon have I not thought about him touching me. Since then I have prayed that it really didn't happen and that possibly I was not as disgusting as I have come to believe. Every day we visited my grandmother's house just a mile from mine. Every time we passed his house, I held my breath, terrified Mom would say something or he might come out. I don't remember a day passing without saying my prayer, "God please, just today let me forget. Let me be like my friends. Please don't let Mommy, John Holt, Bill, Ashley, Mimi, or John think I am bad. Please help them forget. Please God make me forget." I've spent these years hoping that no one would remember, wishing it would be erased from my memory. Everyone did avoid the subject, but I have yet to know a day without thinking about them both, Michael and Trisha, and about how I am this darkened child now. I recall playing with my friends when in the midst of laughing and being little girls, I would suddenly remember. I would try so hard to make the memory of being touched go away, but the nasty feeling they left has never released me.

I can remember trying to talk about it once while Lauren was spending the night. We were in the fourth grade and were suppose to be in bed by eleven. We were desperate to reach the next level on Super Mario Brothers, so we turned down the volume and played well into the night. Lauren's turn was up and, as usual, she rarely died. For some reason my mind kept replaying what had happened between Michael and me. Looking back I know why. I desperately longed for a few moments of purity, a temporary escape from the sordid drama that continued to live in my mind, acting out the events that led me out of innocence, out of my childhood. I remember wishing the tears away at first. But the more I thought about him the more my resistance fell prey to my emotions. I kept telling myself, "You can do this. You can. She will not hate you. She will not think you are weird. Just do it." I hoped she would look at me, and that, seeing the tears, she would have to ask. I sniffled and wiped my eyes, but she didn't notice. I was going to explode. I wanted to tell her. I wanted to know if I was okay. "Lauren, I am different than you, I am not like you."

Her eyes fixed on the video game, she replied. "What are you talking about?"

"I am. I am just different." She really was not responding. I got cold feet and dropped the whole subject. I knew I needed to tell, but how could I explain to another ten-year-old who had only heard of such a horror on TV? I decided to keep my secret between God and me. The knowledge forbidden to a normal innocent child was mine forever. In a moment Michael showed me how my dreams and nightmares could meet. I knew I was different from that afternoon on, and for some reason I never felt worthy of laughing with the freedom, trust, and joy only a child can. I will always pray no one will think I am as awful and disgusting as I began to believe. I promise with all my heart I never wanted it to happen and I didn't mean for it to. If I could have I would have stopped it. I wish Mom, Dad or someone would have fought for me. Are they that embarrassed of me? Are they that ashamed? I didn't want it to happen. I would give anything for that day to have been different, but it won't ever go away. My stomach turns when I think how awful and contaminated everyone must think I am and how weird and different I am from every other girl.

⚬⚬⚬

Well, with every meal today I fought with God's help to keep my head out of the toilet. It would not quit screaming my name and telling me over and over that it holds my relief and happiness. Today was a bad day; I ate too much. The morning will be the true test, with what happens on the scale, followed by the pinch test throughout the day. I hate that I feel that I am losing that powerful little voice that keeps me from eating. I have got to take drastic measures to lose five pounds. I would be perfectly skinny then. Well, tomorrow is a new day, a day of eating right, but it is impossible because I know I have already failed. I love food and despise food.

∞∞

Why don't they realize? Why don't they see that I am not Chelsea anymore? That everyday I become more and more of this disease? My shell validates my identity—my choices, and who I have become. We are so entangled I don't know how to breathe even if I wanted to stand alone. I don't understand. Do they think if they don't talk about it that it will just get better or just go away? Who are they kidding? I mean, this is my life now. It is only in the rarest of times that I know a life outside of my eating disorder. So no, it won't go away. How loud does my body have to scream to make them see that I want out?

∞∞

Over Christmas I was at Lauren's house. Lauren and her sister were talking about a girlfriend of theirs named Elizabeth. She is a few years older than Lauren and I. She had just returned from a treatment center for eating disorders called Remuda Ranch. I was shocked. Elizabeth was always a girl we all looked up to. She had everything to look forward to. Never would I have thought she had an eating disorder, much less need to go to a treatment center. I don't know why I can't stop thinking about her. Her life appeared so flawless. She had everything going for her. She could hide it so well. I, on the other hand, feel like a basket case inside and out. If she had a problem but could hide it so well that she looked perfect on the outside, if she could have this secret life that she could not handle alone, I can't help but think that maybe I might have enough of a problem to go to this place. I would be so humiliated to tell everyone that I had lost control and I needed help. What if they thought I was overreacting or that I was not skinny enough to go? What if they laughed at me and said I needed to deal with this on my own? Why did I have to take this a step further? Had I not gone to the extreme, if I had kept it quiet and kept eating, they never would have known. I could have been the ultimate bulimic. No one would have ever suspected me. I guess in all probability I must not want this for myself or I would have kept on living a secret life.

Going to school today will kill me. I am so miserable it really sucks. I freeze when I go outside. I can't stand the cold.

∞∞

I am miserable. I feel so incredibly fat I don't want to move. I weighed 111 today. My inner thighs are getting bigger by the moment. God please, please I am begging you, don't let me gain weight. As soon as I begin to let myself eat and take a bite with less guilt I gain weight. I love eating. I am obsessed with it. I don't want to leave the house. I will be taken away from food. I can't wait till I get hungry so I can eat. I do not want to go cheer at this basketball game. It will almost kill me to walk through the kitchen without getting a little something to eat. Every step I take I press my legs together as a test. I try so hard to make my inner thighs touch. If they do, I have to take immediate action. Step one is in my head, belittling my every thought and every need. Step two is to continue to press my thighs together to remind myself how I am not good enough and not to think for a second that my body is good.

God, I want to trust you, but when I let go I get fat. My stupid mom got me to go to one of those dumb Alanon meetings. The nerve of her! I think she probably knew they were going to talk about control. She probably told them that control is "my problem." Well I don't care what they say, I am not going to fall for their little tricks.

Made a 4.0 for the semester, I am excited. Please I have got to get back to 105. I don't want any more than that. I don't want to get less than 100 because I hear that girls who get lower than 100 never want to see three digits on the scale again. I hate to think about tomorrow because I just want to go to aerobics and stay home.

∞∞

I have done better today, probably because I weighed 109 this morning. I can't ease up and I still have a ways to go. I ate too many of these fat-free oatmeal cookies. I will probably pay for it tomorrow but I don't feel too guilty. I have got to get up the nerve to tell Mom about Remuda Ranch. The crazy thing is, for the past six months I have been reading from a book called Beyond the Looking Glass, written by patients from the Remuda Ranch Treatment Center.

∞∞

I guess I am oblivious to my body. When I was getting dressed for bed tonight I was so amazed and fascinated with my chest bones. I am so taken with the way they show through my skin. I stood in front of my bathroom mirror for a long time, raising my arms up and down like a bird. I don't know how long I stood there. It was like I was in a trance, watching the thin skin slither over my bones. I can't believe what I have done, my ability to make my body this way. My tiny breasts just hang there because the stuff that once filled them is gone. I did

44

this over and over. I just couldn't believe that I could see every rib and all the breast bones. Wearing these thin white shorts and a bra, I was so impressed with myself that I ran into my parents' room while they were lying in bed. I stood at the foot of the bed and I did the birdlike motion for them, telling them to watch my bones. They looked at me and returned to whatever they were doing. I didn't care. I just said how much I loved it and laughed as I flew out of the room. I am tired and want to go to bed. It really is not that big of a deal.

That is another thing. I hate to have any of my clothes fit too close to my waist. I can't even stand for my underwear to be real fitted. I hate for the elastic to touch my stomach. It is a habitual reminder of how inadequate and unsuccessful I am. Even the elastic has a personality and control over me.

∞∞

I think I might have figured out the source of my weight gain. Those stupid birth control pills. I really don't eat very much, and when I do I throw up. I got really drunk tonight. It doesn't take much. I have always believed in a hell after you die. As horrible as it sounds, I think I have created my hell right here. I am living out my own hell, addicted to hunger pains, shortness of breath, and a screwed-up heart beat. I'm obsessed with picking at my skin, the craving of not eating, the drive to constantly exercise, and with throwing up, but it's never enough. I am starting to believe that I need to go to Remuda Ranch. Maybe I should write Elizabeth and ask her how it is (like it is some amusement park). I go back and forth, loving and hating my life. Never do I enjoy it.

∞∞

You know the physical effects are painful, but feeling and knowing that my soul is dying, dying faster than I know, is even worse. I know it is dying before I ever had a chance to love it. This is not my life. I can't have this problem. It's not a problem. It could develop into one. I really don't care anymore because I would rather die than have someone make me gain weight. I already feel like a failure for not losing more weight. I like to see and feel my bones more than anything. It is more comfort than you know. Going to sleep is difficult. I have always slept on my side, with my knees touching, but the bones hurt so bad that I have to put a pillow between my legs. I can lie in my bed for hours, unable to sleep. I will run my fingers over my frame, convincing myself I am getting fatter. My hip bones are almost sharp; as I rub my palms over my pelvis it's like I am not even touching a body much less my body. The feel of the touch fascinates me. I always tell myself I have got to stop eating so much. Night is sort of like boot camp. I mentally prepare my psyche for the battle, which begins with 6:00 A.M. aerobics.

I have to be here on earth for something more than this—whatever this hell is. How can make a decision about which college I am to go to when I can't even choose what yogurt flavor I want? I have lost interest in everything. I don't care about anything. I don't know anything other than this. But I have to believe that God put me on earth for something other than this. I also have had this feeling that I have to make a move. College is getting closer. I have always thought this would go away before I graduated high school, but it is only a few months away and I am only further in.

∞∞

I am failing. I am getting fatter. I am so repulsed with myself. I just want to go to bed. I say I want to go to bed, but I just lie there. My back has really been messed up lately; I know it's from exercising. I am scared that the doctor might be right; if I don't gain weight I could do enough damage to never be able to have children. I have always dreamed of having a life with kids and a husband, but I can't even leave my house without crying. What has happened? I never wanted it to be like this. I really wish I had the same control that I had three months ago. I would not have dared throw up. Now I have become so desperate that I will do anything.

∞ ∞

I was sitting in the kitchen with Mom. I don't know why or how, but I just started talking. "Um, Mom there is this girl that I went to camp with. She is a few years older than me. She goes to the University of Texas and is a friend of Amy's. Well, Amy and Lauren were telling me that she went to a treatment center for an eating disorder. I mean I never would have thought this girl had a problem in the world. This is the same treatment center who published the devotional book I read everyday. I was thinking maybe we could call this place Remuda Ranch and find out some information about it."

I threw that out, never able to look her in the face. I just stared at our kitchen table waiting for her to tell me that I was overreacting. She didn't say anything. She got up from the table.

"Yes, I need an eight hundred number for a place called Remuda Ranch Treatment Center . . . I think Arizona. Thank you."

I guess she liked the idea. "Wait Mom. Before you call, I really do not want ANYONE to know I am going. I think I will tell people I am going to visit Dad and be gone for awhile. I probably won't have to be gone very long anyway."

She calmly said, "We will work out the details later. Do you want to call or do you want me to?"

We had taken this conversation up to my room; the kitchen was too cold. Squirming on my bed with my head in the pillow

I said, "You call. I am not talking to them. I wouldn't have a clue what to say."

Mom called and I got a note pad. Vigorously I wrote down questions for her to ask.

Finally she got sick of it and said, "She is right here. I will let you talk to her."

The soothing voice on the other end was as comforting to hear as this call could be. She did most of the talking, explaining the process of being admitted, and she told me they would send me information and a video. Our task was to talk to the insurance company and find out all the information. The major task for me would be to tell Dad. How was I going to tell him? He doesn't have a clue what has gone on.

The last time we talked about it was in November when he, Ashley, and I went to buy jeans. I have to give my sister credit. She has never been afraid to call my problem by name, and more or less blatantly pointed out to Dad that my jeans were tiny. Walking through the store she loudly said, "Dad, Dad, this is not normal. Do you see that these are size 3 jeans? These are for little girls. And they are baggy on her." I smiled, soaking up the feelings of success that came with size three Levi's being loose now. Anyway, when the conversation with Remuda ended, I began to cry. What have I gotten myself into?

∞∞

Everything is good to go with Remuda. I plan to tell people and not hide that I am going. I have my assessment in three days. I am getting scared. I don't know if this is what I really need and want. They have this thing called family week. Imagine my whole family there: John Holt, Ashley, Bill, Jude, Mom, and Dad.

I want to kill food. I want to rip it, stab it, and beat it. What will people think when I return? Will I have any friends?

Will people still associate with me? Will they still love me? I feel guilty because I have not been a friend to anyone. I am really lucky and blessed to have so many friends that love me and still will be loyal enough to stick by me. I can't imagine being a friend with someone as awful as me or as boring. I miss so much school but I just can't do it now. I have missed some days lately. I hope that God and I will reunite up in Arizona. I threw up badly for a few days but I didn't today.

∞∞

Once again my evening visit to the kitchen. As usual it followed the hour-and-a-half dinner and dessert I'd had and then threw up. I talked to Remuda today for my two-hour assessment. They had tons of questions for me to answer. I have been so afraid that they would think I wasn't sick enough or that I was really making a big deal out of nothing. I hadn't thrown up for a day, but today I really hit rock bottom.

∞∞

Why do I do this? I make commitments because I hate saying no but cannot even fathom the thought of going through with the plans. The thought of leaving my house to do something other than exercise or go to school makes me ill. I don't think my sister is comfortable with coming to Remuda. Maybe God knows best. School was good today, maybe because I went to 6:00 A.M. aerobics and that got me started on the right foot. I haven't talked to Dad for two weeks. I guess that is not all that strange. I got some new clothes today. Shopping is the biggest chore. It takes me so long to decide on anything. I just don't feel like I really deserve new clothes. Besides, what if I choose something and I don't wear it or it is not just right? I always leave the tags on the clothes, let them sit in my closet awhile, and then return them. I convince myself I don't deserve them. Today I really hated myself. I felt fat and worthless. I must lose five pounds. I don't look anorexic at all. It is such a joke that someone could think I am.

⚮⚮

I just love to cook, but I never eat what I cook. Well, except for the fat-free cake batter. I eat that and I just can't stop. I also love to cook these pizzas that have tons of vegetables on top with very little crust. I never eat the crust, just the vegetables on top. I also love tomatoes and broccoli. I could eat that all day. If I make a tomato sauce I use big chunks of tomatoes and lots of veggies, then put it on pasta but never eat the pasta. Well, maybe on a good day I will have a little bite of pasta.

Some foods I just can't control myself around. Like this chocolate pudding or the fat-free cake batter. I eat so much and just can't get enough and then I throw up. Like tonight, I just kept throwing up and throwing up. Then I'd go eat and throw up again. I dry heave but still I make myself do it again. I know there is more stuff down there. I have all these little scratches on my knuckles from my teeth scrapping across my hand. They hurt really bad and my hands are all red. I like to throw up in the downstairs bathroom because it is the best at not getting clogged. After throwing up I put a mud mask on my face to take the puffiness out. I am so scared. My parents are going to a party and I am going to be all alone. I can't control myself when I know I am alone. I don't want to throw up or spit food out. It hurts so bad, but I don't know what else to do. It is like I am sinking in quicksand and no one even knows I am lost. I am so ashamed that I throw up. How disgusting. But when I do it, I don't realize that I am really doing it, if that makes any sense. It's like I am so unaware of anything inside me or outside. Almost as though I am not even myself. I want to go cook, and I need to be at aerobics because it scares me that I am not. If I was really good at my job, I would be doing aerobics.

∽∽

I leave today. I don't remember ever throwing up my breakfast before, but knowing it would be my last time to choose, I had no choice. I ran to the mirror—I wanted to make one last attempt to see myself the way others saw me, but the emptiness that consumes me has made it too difficult to see. I am terrified—I knew this could never last. Either it would go or I would go with it. It is sort of like holding your breath, something eventually would have to blow.

# Innocence Stolen

*C*helsea *was almost four. She was a precocious, precious, innocent bundle of joy with a head full of blond curls and a contagious personality. She would swing under the oak trees in Mimi's front yard and play with the adoring, patient, older neighborhood children who included her in their outdoor games. They were especially caring and protective of Chelsea when John Holt and Ashley weren't there to watch over her. Mimi's yard, kitchen, and family room had a constant flow of children of all ages (seven to sixteen years) when school was out.*

*It was a summer afternoon when I drove to pick up Chelsea at my parent's home. Mimi told me she had given Chelsea permission to play across the street in the home of a woman whom I'll call Ann. I had known Ann since I was a teenager, having grown up just a block away. She had two sons; one of them was Michael, who at sixteen was the oldest of the group of kids on the block. He and his younger brother had always been exceptionally nice to Chelsea.*

*I walked across the street to Ann's house to fetch Chelsea. In my memory it happened something like this.*

*"Hi, Ann. Mimi said Chelsea's here playing with the boys. Thanks for having her over." Ann complimented Chelsea. "She is so cute. The boys just adore her. She's downstairs in*

*Michael's room." Ann turned at the top of the stairs and called politely, "Michael, Chelsea's mom is here. Send Chelsea up here." Chelsea came trotting up the stairs, or walking slowly— I don't remember. I'm sure I gave her a hug and probably picked her up, which I still did, not because she needed to be carried but because I loved to hold her. I'm sure I would have uttered something like, "Thanks, Ann, and tell Michael thank you, too. Bye now."*

*As we walked to the car I would have told Chelsea that we were going home where Ashley and John Holt were waiting for us and then asked her, "Did you have fun, honey? What did you all do?" By now we were getting into the car. I had barely started driving when Chelsea's little voice began to unfold an experience no parent is ever prepared to hear. Her voice was always deep for her age, soft and rarely as serious as when she stated a profound truth for her. "Michael is not nice. I don't like Michael any more. I don't like him, Mom."*

*Chelsea had my attention. I heard the seriousness in her tone. Her simple statement alerted me. My protective radar was up, yet I asked calmly, "What happened? What did Michael do?"*

*Her little words fell across me in that car like shards of glass. I wanted the words to stop, but I knew I had to encourage their tumbling out. Most of all I had to remain calm and not scare her with my reaction as she tried to tell me, "Mom, Michael showed me his penis. It was big with hair all around it. He laid on me. He pulled off my panties. He put his penis on me. He did things I do not like. I don't ever want to go over there again. I'm never going to play with him again."*

*Known for always having the words to console, I found myself at a loss. My mind was swirling. Thoughts crossed on top of one another in less than a few seconds, "Don't panic. Whom do I call? Speak softly. Reassure her. Don't cry. Don't scare her.*

*Breathe. Should I go back to Michael's house. No! Never! Get Chelsea to safety. Take her home. Tell her it's not her fault. Say something about how Michael is bad. God, help me say the right thing. I hate him. I want to hurt him. Help. Tell Mimi. How can I. Call Holt? Get home. Don't panic."*

*What I said in the quietest, controlled voice I could muster was, "Chelsea, I love you. I am sorry Michael did that. He was bad and very wrong to do that to you. You did nothing wrong. I am so glad you told me. Thank you for telling me. You are right, you will never go over there again. I don't like Michael either. Michael is mean. We're going to go home. Thank you, sweetheart, for telling me. I love you. I am very mad at Michael. Did he hurt you? Does anything hurt?"*

*We had only about four or five blocks to drive. As we were pulling into our drive, Chelsea answered, "No, Michael did not hurt me, but I didn't want him to do that. I hate Michael."*

*When we walked in the kitchen, either John Holt, who was eleven then, grabbed his little sister, or she ran full force for him. He had become her surrogate father. There was a mutual admiration society going on between them. They would hug, kiss, and tease then start all over again. It was no different that day, but everything was different. John Holt just didn't know it. I knew I had to tell John Holt. He had to know. I needed him to know. I needed his loving her. I needed him to share my anger. I needed John Holt. He was always there for me, for Chelsea. She was the most precious thing in his life. He would be her protector again.*

*He was only eleven—the size of a fifteen-year-old—but only eleven. I was wrong to need him so much. I hadn't parentified him, but I had allowed him frequently to take on the father role where Chelsea was concerned. He was a natural. When we brought her home from the hospital, he would just stand quietly at the side of her crib and watch over her for the longest time. He would never wake her. He might reach in and touch her hand as she slept, letting her chubby fingers wrap around his big-brother seven-year-old finger. He couldn't wait for her to wake up, but he always did. He had all the patience in the world for her and he still does. To rock her was his greatest pleasure. One of my favorite photographs is of John Holt hugging Chelsea, squeezing her stomach as he chanted "Chubby, chubby" as she giggled with joy. The saddest picture I have is of Chelsea at seventeen, crying with her head resting on John Holt's chest, held by his huge, tender hand. If I hadn't nursed her, he would have loved giving her a bottle—anything to be near her, to nurture her, to love her. How could I tell him? I had to tell him.*

*Ashley, my thirteen-year-old firstborn, was in the kitchen as well. Where John Holt was the quiet, gentle child, Ashley was the strong, confrontational, exuberant adolescent. She came out of my womb with more spirit than I was prepared for, a mind that was leaps ahead of me, and more energy than all of us put together. Ashley knew me well, and she had a firstborn's intuition that told her when things weren't quite right. She also would not tolerate unanswered questions. Today was no different. Immediately Ashley sought out the cause of my appearance. "Mom, you look like you've seen a ghost. What's wrong? Where have you been? Did something happen?"*

*The questions kept coming. What they were, or how I got Chelsea out of the room, I don't recall. I'm sure I knew then that Ashley would not be put off for long. She never took excuses or ruses well. She is too bright to accept trite answers that don't match with behavior and body language.*

*Recently Ashley has confirmed my memory of that day. She remembers knowing something was seriously wrong the moment she saw me. She also reassures me that the answers to her questions did not come till after Chelsea was out of hearing distance. We both assume I escorted Chelsea upstairs to watch television in my room, with some transparent excuse to Ashley meant to assure her that nothing was wrong. I probably tried to communicate to Ashley by darting my eyes toward Chelsea to indicate that the discussion shouldn't be held in front of her.*

*Now I had to tell John Holt and Ashley. They had been through so much with me. The divorce and their father's move to Los Angeles had left scars. We had been married thirteen years. When their father met and married a Hollywood celebrity, the children had had to endure the celebrity publicity, People magazine, and TV shows that accompanied the marriage. While John Holt had provided much of the play and nurturing in Chelsea's rearing, Ashley had been called on for the more responsible duties a sister nine years older can perform to help out an overwhelmed single mother. John Holt and Ashley would respond to the crisis differently because they had unique personalities and different relationships with Chelsea. But more than anything, what the three of us had in common that afternoon was that we had worked as a team to raise and care for Chelsea. The bottom line is that we loved her. She had been sexually assaulted and they had to know.*

*I feel sure that before I returned to John Holt and Ashley I physically examined Chelsea, but I have no recollection of what I said to reassure her or to explain what I was looking for. I probably said something to make it sound like checking her out was no big deal, but I just wanted to make sure Michael had not hurt her. I probably asked for more information as I did this. All this has been suppressed in my memory, but I know I realized that the call I would be making soon to her pediatrician would require me to know whether she had been physically hurt. There was no tearing or bleeding, so I probably hid my anxiety with comforting words meant to reassure Chelsea that everything would be okay. Settling her on my bed with a favorite TV show, I returned downstairs to her waiting brother and sister.*

*I have asked Ashley and John Holt what they remember me saying. Like me, they do not remember the exact words, but they both have the same overall recollection that I gave cursory details such as, "Chelsea was playing with Michael when I picked her up. When she got in the car, she told me he had exposed himself, took off her panties and laid down on her."*

*John Holt hit the table and yelled as he shot out of his chair, "I'm going to kill him!"*

*Ashley was standing by the sink and screamed, "That filthy bastard. How could he do that to her? Did he rape her?"*

*I told them I had examined Chelsea, and I quoted some of her wording for what had happened, explaining, "There is no way she would have understood what he did to her, but her instincts told her Michael was bad. She's never seen the things she described. For sure he has sexually abused her."*

*The correct terminology today would be "sexual assault." But remember, I worked at a child abuse prevention agency and I knew about sexual abuse. I was to find out that I did not then know the best approach for handling such an incident, and neither did any of the professionals I consulted with on that day seventeen years ago. Therein lies the next tragedy.*

*Now it was time for me to calm down Ashley and John Holt so Chelsea would not hear their horror. I explained, and cautioned Ashley, who was saying she would tell everyone at his school what a pervert he was. John Holt needed to be stopped from going over to Michael's house to beat him up or do something worse. I redirected their focus from Michael to Chelsea. "Our concern is for Chelsea. It is imperative that she not feel that she did something wrong. If she sees how upset you are or hears your angry voices, she'll be frightened and think she has done something wrong. We must be calm and not make this sound like the crisis it is."*

*"Well, what are you going to do? What can we do? I still think we should do something to Michael," Ashley protested as John Holt became quiet.*

*"I need some advice. I'm going to call Dr. Nyman. He may need to see her. I also want to call the Parenting Guidance Center. This is what their therapists are specialists at. Then I will call your dad. He has to know, but I want to have some answers first before I call him."*

*"Someone has got to do something about Michael," said Ashley. "What if he tries to hurt her again? What if he does something to some other little girl? There're four little girls living on that block. Their parents need to be warned. Mom, Michael is evil. He is so gross." The more Ashley lashed out, the more John Holt withdrew into his private pain.*

*Luckily I reached Dr. Nyman, the children's pediatrician, that afternoon. He thought he was reassuring me by saying this was not that uncommon. Adolescent boys often acted out sexually with someone younger, he explained. He advised me not to make a big deal about it. He believed I could traumatize her more by showing my anger. Moreover, he continued, we should just go on as if nothing had happened. He felt she was probably so young she would not remember the incident. Dr. Nyman was in his late fifties and what he was advising me was what was being taught and practiced at the time. If this had happened just a few years later, I'm sure his advice would have been very different and much more therapeutically healing. Thank goodness, much was to be learned by the mental health professionals and physicians. But for now, for Chelsea their answers were wrong. More than unhelpful, they were even hurtful as the years to come would prove.*

*Reassured and having been directed to do nothing, I sought confirmation from the place I worked, from the people I believed knew what was best. I quickly reached the clinical director of the Parenting Guidance Center. He knew more about child abuse than just about anyone in the state if not the nation. He had worked his way up through the County Child Protective Services. He was a highly respected therapist and supervisor of other therapists. Like Dr. Nyman, he believed Chelsea would probably not remember the incident if we did not overreact and alarm her. He did suggest that I not drop the subject but to encourage her gently to express her feelings of anger, fear, and whatever else she was trying to deal with. The director also said I should make statements that would relieve her of any guilt or feelings of being bad, and restate what I had said about Michael being bad, the guilty person who had wronged her. He also instructed me to ask her whether she had any questions and answer them as simply and honestly as I could. Of course he was there for me not only that afternoon but also in the days following, when I needed someone professional to process what had happened and how I was feeling.*

*I must digress briefly here. The Parenting Guidance Center was the first agency in the United States to address the problems of parenting and child abuse in a comprehensive way, providing education, family and individual counseling in Tarrant County, and preventative programs in the Fort Worth school district. It utilized both an excellent professional staff and a highly trained core of volunteers. However, play therapy was new and was not a part of what was available at the center. Within a year or two it was introduced and became an essential part of the treatment for the youngest victims of child abuse. Play therapy is a perfect medium for a child to work out his or her feelings. Sometimes a child who is not comfortable or not verbally capable of talking about their abuse can act out the incident with anatomically correct dolls or tell their story through drawings. The benefits of play therapy for an abused child can be tremendous, because by helping the child communicate about the abuse, it can minimize the psy-*

*chological effects of repressed memory or inappropriate assumption of guilt or shame.*

*Over the following days I tried to relieve Chelsea of any feelings of guilt or shame when we daily drove by Michael's house on the way to her grandparents' home. I would speak of how I was mad at Michael for hurting her and how Michael was bad for treating her in a scary way. Chelsea would agree with her soft voice saying, "I'm never going to Michael's again." After a while she did not say anything and I stopped mentioning it, hoping the professionals were right that she would probably forget it. My advisers were wrong. She never forgot. The shame was like cancer eating at her precious mind. Little did I know she thought about it every day from that day on.*

*I made other necessary calls that day to her father in Los Angeles, to a few of my best friends, to her grandparents, to Bill, the wonderful man I would marry the following year, and last of all to Michael's mother, Ann. I remember that call in more detail than all the others. I told Ann in the most direct and simple words I could muster what Michael had done to Chelsea. I also repeated some of the words Chelsea had used to describe the assault. Ann agreed that Chelsea could not have made up the story. She said that she believed Chelsea and that she was very sorry. I told her that Michael needed professional help before someone else was assaulted. She agreed and said she would find a therapist immediately. To this day I do not know how Ann dealt with Michael. Michael kept a low profile. I never saw him playing on the block with the younger children. I would see his car parked in front of his house. He graduated from high school two years later and left for college. He is married now and lives in another Texas city. I am sorry to say he is a father now—a very scary thought.*

# Part Two:
# Spring 1994—A Spring of Hope

༄ ༅

*As is the inner, so is the outer.*
—GNOSTIC AXIOM

# Letters to My Mother

For a moment I believe and for a moment I might know.
Then forget what I know, and try to retrieve what was
    meant to be.
How can I go on and not believe? Once more is all I plead.
If I go away will *it* go away? Or if I hide maybe I won't
    hear the little whispers in my ear.
Why do I wonder if there is more? Why have I begun this
    desire to change?
It would be so much simpler if I would just believe and
    laugh at the blindness of tomorrow.

∽∾

*February 15, 1994*
Dear Mom,

The pain that now consumes me is far greater than any I could have dared to dream. The darkness is more present than any I have known. I believe that I have felt as much pain as my soul can bear. I was so strong till I got to the ranch and a woman showed me the grounds where I would live for the next couple of months. The tour made the reality that I am here hit hard. Then I could not stop crying. All I kept thinking about is how much I miss my friends. I can honestly say I would give my life to be in your lap for five minutes with you constantly hugging me and kissing me. I have come up with so many fears. I have now convinced myself that I am going to fail out of school or never be able to keep up when I return. I am scared to death you all are going to forget me. Five weeks just pounds my every thought. I really wanted to call and get a pep talk.

I was lying virtually naked in the doctor's office, crying my eyes out. I begged God to send the Holy Spirit to be with me to help the pain and to guide me. They have locks on the scales, and they hid my weight from me, then took two huge tubes of blood. They said my EKG looked good. Anything positive gives me hope that I will get out of here sooner. I am really pissed that I have given three years to this bullshit. The girls are nice, skinny, and some gross. I don't want to be like them! I am going to use this time to put an end to this crap. I wish you would think about coming to visit early or something. I am in the main lodge with three other girls in my room. I will get out of my room faster than anyone (which indicates I am making progress).

I wish I could describe to you how painful it is to be away from everyone I love so much and everything I like and know. I think God has helped me realize that not much was going to change at home, but here I will get the old Chelsea back, only stronger. I won't forget or abandon all I know—my friends and family—but just strengthen all that love. I am tired of having a problem. I want it gone. I want to be healthy.

Well, it has been a few hours since I wrote and I met with the doctor. He said the enamel on my teeth was starting to come off from the bile in my mouth after I throw up. I also had dinner. They fix the plates for you and have your name on it, and I ate my whole dinner. I want to advance as fast as I can. I am absolutely miserable right now. You have no idea how homesick I am. I love you more than life itself. I need to go because I have all these bubble tests to take. Mother, I am so scared about school. It seems so overwhelming. Writing is making me more sad. I feel like this time here will be an eternity. I love you with everything inside, and it kills me, the pain I feel without you near.

∞∞

*February 16, 1994*
Dear Mom,

This morning I was awakened at 6:00 A.M. by the nurse taking my roommates' vital signs. Then she took mine. After that I got completely nude (except for the paper sheath), and I went to the nurses' station to be weighed. I step on the scale backward and the nurse reads the scale. Outside it looks like night the sky is so dark. I am now at level 1A. If my blood work is okay when it gets back from the lab, I move to level 1B. At the first level they treat everyone the same. We are driven everywhere and do nothing for ourselves. They don't want any physical strain until the test results come back. It is pretty silly for them to think I might keel over. The only reason that would happen is that it is so hot. This is a cute place. The kitchen is really homelike, with these six-person wood tables (it reminds me of the old Facts of Life TV show). A nurse sits at the end of each table and eats her meal with you. We cannot flush the toilet without having it checked by the nurse, even though she stands in there with you while you go to the bathroom. Thank goodness I don't have to really go to the bathroom yet. You also have to wait thirty minutes after meals before you can go to your room. Everyone is so nice. They want to hug you all the time, and they are so proud of me because it was my choice to come and I want so badly to get better. During meals, we have to roll up our sleeves and keep our hands on top of the table. They are really calm about everything and are not mean at all.

I love to go to meal times because I had forgotten how real food tastes. I'd also forgotten that it is okay for me to have a meal, much less a meal with fat in it. I am not afraid to eat because I trust that they won't let me get fat.

I really do like food, although I have been experiencing a lot of pain in my stomach after I eat because I get so full. I feel very nourished. We must eat everything on our plate and drink all our juice. If we don't they just make up the calories with Ensure. I had a huge piece of French toast with syrup, cottage cheese, and an apple for breakfast. I get to eat ground beef, eggs, steak, and peanut butter, and I don't have to worry because they have it all figured out in my meal plan and calorie intake. Every morning we have chapel, and I love it. I am relieved to be here. I have made a commitment not to screw around because the staff is not going to do it for me. The more I resist the change, the longer my life waits to regain normalcy. I believe that I will get my life back, but this experience is far more painful than anything the world I left could have prepared me for. I am beginning to understand what being broken is all about. I just can't describe the freedom of not fearing every bite that approaches my mouth and betting my life that the next bite will be the one that will make or break my self-worth. My greatest fear is that everyone will abandon me, and I just love everyone so much. I don't want to lose anyone close to me.

∽◌∾

*February 17, 1994*
Dear Mom,
There is this new girl and she is awful. Everyone hates her. She makes it so hard for all the girls to eat because she throws her plate off the table, pitches fits, and even has thrown her plate on the wall. Then she talks constantly about how fattening and disgusting the food is, (which is the kiss of death for any

person trying to recover from an eating disorder at the dinner table). You all would be so proud of me. I am not letting her get to me, and I have been really strong and dealt with things that I have been running from for so long.

Mom, I want you to think about what came out in group today: I am angry at you for being a victim of my disease. I for so long have protected you in every way I knew how, and trying to be the perfect child is killing me. I hate that I got that message or chose that role because I am realizing how sick that has made me. This is hard to tell you because I never want to hurt you.

I have asked to get back on birth control, but the doctor wants to see if my body can get back on its cycle without the pill. Please think about what I have said. I love you very much.

P.S. I also think my disorder has to do with performing.

❦

*February 18, 1994*
Dear Mom,

I won't write much since I will talk with you tomorrow. I had a hard day today. My emotions and feelings are so alive. I really thought of giving up today. I'm realizing how alone I am and that no one can fight for my recovery but me. This is my life and it is up to me now, at eighteen, to choose whether I want to fight for a life other than the hell I was living. Attempting to conceptualize my mortality or living a full life is exhausting. I can't expect you, or anyone for that matter, to understand this or to begin to know what to say or how to help. If I want my life back, I believe I can find it here. I just have to believe in myself and hold on to the hope God has never let me loose.

I have probed my body for resources it did not possess. I

was turning to my body to change something it wasn't capable of changing. My actions only allowed me to continue living the secrets that consumed me, only strengthening my connection to the shaming memories.

I was very overwhelmed at the end of the day. I didn't want to do it alone (recovery, facing life). The ranch is beautiful. There is a place on the property where green grass covers a large hill. After my classes today I felt so lost and burnt out. I went out on this hill where I could be alone, and I just buried my head in the grass and began to cry. As I was crying, I began talking to God, asking him over and over if I was doing what he wanted. I prayed so hard that I would not have to recover all alone. I needed more than anything to know that I was on the right track, that I was right where he wanted me. Most of all, I wanted to not face this alone. Well, as I continued to say this type of stuff, I found this fear and even anger inside of me that was so intense. It came from being so terrified of being alone, and it was growing stronger and stronger.

Never before had I seen black Labradors on the ranch, and you know how passionate I am about black Labs. While I had my face buried in the cold grass, crying my eyes out, two black Labs came barreling on top of me, licking me profusely. They stayed and continued to play around me and with me. Without my consent my tears became tears of joy. I realized in those moments that God is pleased with me and that he loves me and wants me right where I am. Most of all I will believe from this day on that I will never be alone in my recovery. Never again will I doubt God's presence and his support of my recovery. We are going to kick butt together. I am so blessed that God is on my side.

Thanks so much for the flowers you and Bill sent me. It meant a lot. I get so tired here because I feel so much and cry all the time. It is absolutely exhausting. There are so many new girls coming that I feel like I am a veteran. I am floored that I have been here a week. I have been having some crazy dreams despite my troubled sleep.

The letter you sent me from University of Texas says that I will be put off till April for review. Great. If they don't accept me, where will I go?

I have moved out of the main house and down to the cabanas. My old roommate couldn't move in with me because she was unable to advance into level 2, due to her poor physical health. My therapist sort of bugs me. I am afraid that I might be able to trick her or that she might not catch everything that I need to deal with. But she could make me eat my words next week.

I have the most incredible roommate. Her name is Grey. She is the best. She is a year younger than I, but we really have a good time together.

In a week I have to write and read my life story to the women who are in group therapy with me. My group consists of eight women and two therapists. I have to tell everything. I mean every breath I took that I can recall, starting with me in your womb—a little strange.

They have these staff meetings here that piss me off. They all get together and compare notes about me. It's the whole damn staff. They watch everything—every action, expression, or statement. They relate each observation to your program and progress. They await any insight I might unconsciously reveal.

We have leisure activities here. They are to remind us of some of the fun things we used to do that our disease has taken us away from, stuff that we might not have had time for because we were too wrapped up in feeding the addiction. For example, today we jumped rope and hula-hooped. Some of the girls get into trouble or are told to calm down because they just start spinning and jumping and won't slow down. I guess they think they can burn some calories without the staff realizing it. Right! Did you know that you need only two hours of exercise a week to be healthy? Any more than that you are doing for reasons other than your health. Less exercise time will really give me a lot more time for my day.

Well, I am very tired since we get up at 6:00 A.M. I better go to bed. And if you talk to my therapist, don't be nice to her. She started talking about our relationship in group. She keeps using this word "enmeshed." I hate the way it sounds. It has something to do with you and me being too attached. Hearing her talk about you at all makes me cry, but for her to say outright that we are not good for each other put me over the edge. I guess they know best, but it still made me mad. I love you so much!

Love,
Chelsea

～～～

*February 19, 1994*
Dear Mom,

I am so excited that I am really going to get better. After crying, I felt for a short time the old me. I am so happy and I feel a sense of peace for the person I am discovering. I am starting to like myself. Fulfilled is a feeling I never knew could exist inside of me. I definitely want to reserve the right to write a letter the next day that is not a joyous one. I can't believe all my revelations in just twenty-four hours. You have no idea how hard they have you work on yourself, repairing and dealing with stuff—your past and present unmarked feelings. I don't like that I can't talk to anyone at home for a week. It's like the staff in their little meetings have decided that I may not be doing as well as I think I am. Privileges and freedom are what make this place tick. But I know that every minute I am here (despite my limitations and their rules) God and I grow closer. I don't want anyone back home to forget about me. I am in control of my recovery. Even though I can't talk on the phone I am getting better. Well that's all for now. Sorry I got a little random. I will write more letters later.

Mom, I love you so much. Please don't stop loving me. I mean that. It scares me. I am scared to hear about all the stuff that has been going on at school. I know people are talking about me like I am some freak. I can't bear to think of all the homework I am missing.

I have never felt so loved. I can't even tell you how many people write me. Each one gives me more courage and belief that maybe I don't see myself or perceive the situation accurately. All the nurses say I get the award for the most mail any patient has received. I just feel bad because I don't have a lot of time to write everyone back, but I will work it out.

ᢙᢙ

*February 20, 1994*
Dear Mom,

Yesterday I had Body Image class. I began talking about my fear of accepting and liking my body, however God made it. My fear of loving and accepting my body would mean giving up my ideals of a perfect body, as well as the whole facade, the rituals I have engaged in the past two and a half years. I wonder what or whose life I have been trying to create. I know I had no place trying to live that life out. When I gain weight and accept it, I will still feel like a failure. My gross behavior and my grave attempts to make the pain go away were efforts to reach perfection. When your purpose in life is to be perfect, drastically changing that ideal is bound to be devastating. I am told my fear is normal.

Looking into all these areas helps me realize my craving for control—control that I thought I had, although I never did and never will. Yesterday I made a decision to put only good and healthy thoughts in my mind because I do want to start loving my body! Unless I start telling myself good things I will never start to see, feel, or believe they are so. I was really killing myself trying so hard to be the perfect girl. Believing that it's not my duty to sacrifice my happiness for others is so foreign to my way of logic. But I can't and won't have that be my job anymore.

The weird part is that I never received compliments when I was so thin, but I kept on. My eating disorder brought nothing but pain to those around me, but I kept on. I really believed that if the outside was perfect the inside would be also. I would have bet a million dollars that every girl I thought was beautiful, with her perfect body, had a perfect life. I mean really, what more could she want? If they are so incredibly beautiful how could anything be wrong in their lives?

Well, I am finding out that beauty doesn't dictate what life gives you. For the rest of my life I am going to be on an adventure, discovering why I am here in the world, what my purpose is, and best of all, to find out who I am without an eating disorder. Now that I am not going to have a life that I cope with through an addiction, I have choices—choices to fill the huge space in myself and my heart with whatever I want. It will be a process of really learning and believing the pure truth that the only way I will ever live out my life will be working from the inside out. Continually I will tell myself that I am not a number on a scale or a size in a piece of clothing. I am Chelsea above whatever else I choose to be, and I am not defined by my body, my appearance, or a number.

It is great to know that all my dehydrated organs have been replenished. All that matters is my health. I've realized that throughout life I will be confronted by people with potentially destructive comments and assumptions. These opinions are only given power if I give power to them. Their weight is defined by my perception. I realize that another's words or opinions are not about me but a reflection of their perspective and their experiences in the world and in themselves. It will be my choice whether I take on their thoughts as truth or have the courage to find my own. I have been told how hard returning to the real world will be, how hard it will be not to get sucked back in—as though I don't know. As problems arise, they tell me to get a reality check from a person whom I trust, to consider the source, and then to decide whether the words fit into my life. Most important, I need to remember that a person's perception is not indicative of the world's perception.

It's hard to know who you are at all times. I don't think it is possible to always know. I guess like right now, when I am redefining myself and everything in my life is focused on getting better, understanding my feelings is much simpler. In the real world it will be up to me to search and value my feelings as they come. When I neglect to respond to or acknowledge my feelings, I am more vulnerable to others' actions and susceptible to their influence. Maybe that is one reason I find myself so empty. I don't have a clue about me, only them and what makes them happy. "They" know what I "should" do with my life. I make choices from "I should." I don't acknowledge what I need or want. I simply assume "they" know what is best.

I have an assignment to write down all the stuff that I like and don't like, my beliefs, morals, strengths, weaknesses, and most of all, my goals for my life. This assignment is to help me realize what has been inside all this time but has been smothered by my desire to do my life perfectly, which no one can do (I take a deep breath every time I say that). They love to give assignments here.

I had Art Therapy today. With our eyes closed we were to imagine the most peaceful and joyous place to us. Then we were to draw what we saw, who we took with us, and to describe whether music was playing and the way things smelled. Mine was so beautiful, with green grass everywhere, the bluest water, chubby cherubs with golden curls flying around, chubby puppy Labradors, fields of tulips, cool bright green grass, and huge willow trees. The music is always in harmony with the running waterfall. The cherubs would take my hand and I would fly with them. Sometimes I would sit and watch them, and sometimes I would dance with them. My world was love and it was joy. I can go there in my mind anytime I need to. I will always be close to my heart there. My drawing wasn't all that bad either.

Please save this letter so you can show me the truth if I start to lose my way. I am also going to ask you guys to take my scale and throw it away. I am not that scale and I am so FUCK-ING sick of letting my self-worth and life revolve around it. Burn that son of a bitch. Just burn it! Thank God! It feels great to say good-bye to one of my biggest controllers.

I love you all,
Chelsea

# Remuda Ranch

I figure the best way to begin my day is with God. I want to start writing in the morning to help me do just that. I am so excited about the new thoughts, ideas, and feelings the Lord has given me. God, I want to put my recovery in your control because when I tried to do it my way, well . . . you can see where that got me. I have this confusion: the paradox of giving up control, letting go, and in turn regaining order in my life. God, please help me every step of the way and show me where you want me. I don't want my life to be about this uncontrollable addiction. I have the hardest time calling myself an addict. I have pegged an addict with a negative connotation. I can't bear to think of myself in the terms of an addict. I hate that word. It is like that feeling when you watch a sex scene with your grandparents. You just think "yuck, not now." I can't bear to hear "addict" and "Chelsea" in the same breath.

⏤∞⏤

Yesterday was awesome! I did it. I told my life story to the group. I told everything. I started off reading my story staring at my paper, but the therapist asked me to look up and see the faces of everyone staring at me. My neck was so heavy I could hardly raise it. As I looked up all I could see was my heart on a cutting board awaiting the butcher's cleaver. I decided when I came here that hiding the truth or lying to anyone would only prolong my getting a life back. Besides the secrets I told today had to come out. The secrets were toxic. I knew my greatest secret was a detailed description of my being sexually abused. I felt my life, my pride, and the shame that had consumed me for twelve years was just dangling in the middle of this circle of women. They asked me again to raise my head while telling each vivid detail. I physically could not. I was so ashamed of how disgusting I had been made since that day. I was so sure I would not have a friend in the world once they knew the truth about my disgusting life. Slowly my eyes began to rise from the dirt on the ground. Their eyes loved me and accepted me in a way their words never could.

The group talked about my belief that they would stone me before they would welcome me. They were shocked that I would feel so horrible about myself, especially when I was only four. Both situations were out of my control. I feel free.

Later that afternoon I met with my therapist, Amy. We began a series of sessions discussing the abuse and working through it. Walking back from the circle of women, I felt something I never knew I had the right to feel: it was not my fault and I am not the one to blame. Today I was more alive and more free than I could ever tell. I am so grateful to you Lord for the relief I feel and courage you gave me to tell what happened. I guess you really will make good out of the bad. It is an amazing feeling to reveal to all those people every secret I have ever known and still to be loved. I feel like I could fly.

∞∞

*And God is faithful; He will not lead you to be tempted beyond what you can bear. But when you are tempted, He will also provide a way out so you can stand up under it.*
—1 Corinthians 10:13

Help me slow down and look around at all you are doing for me. I am the luckiest girl in the world. I love that verse and I know my recovery is dependent on it.

> *With favor You will surround me with a shield.*
> —Psalms 5:12

∽

I am coming to understand why my therapist wants my relationship to change between Mom and me. The way we have been functioning—especially toward the end—is horrible for both of us. They use this stupid word all the time, "enmeshed." But it makes sense that we are too dependent on one another, that we don't live our lives for ourselves. We are too involved with each other. I am seeing that this is a common thread between mothers and daughters, especially in those who have eating disorders. I think the pressure of being responsible for another's mental well-being is far too great—especially for a child to assume that obligation for her parent. I love her so much, but I need to let her go so that I can grow for myself. I want my own life, and I trust she will be fine no matter what I do. To think that I alone can have control over another is really prideful and even self-centered. I am grateful I don't have that kind of control. Look where that belief has taken me, the things it has led me to tell myself: "If I can be a little skinnier, or not eat the whole piece of toast everything will be okay." "If she is not happy or if I can't make him laugh then I really don't deserve to eat." God, I don't want to do this alone and I know that you will take care of my family in a more productive way than I ever could. I want to work as hard as I can and deal with all I can. I want my life and I want this chance to live.

I can hardly wait. The whole family is coming this week,

except for my sister, Ashley. I have to assume Ashley knows what is best. Where do I start? How will I even begin to explain this to my family? I know that sometime between fifteen and sixteen I started my eating disorder. Now, at eighteen, I am saddened by the years lost to my preoccupation with my diet and body. As a result I have missed so much of a normal teenage life. When you devote your life to something, it seems almost impossible to not have your self-worth and self-esteem wrapped up in it. My surrendering has left me with little self-esteem. How can I trust myself when I choose to stick my fingers down my throat and starve myself in some bizarre unconscious suicide attempt?

Fear fuels my insane drive for perfection. Deep down I know I can never attain my high expectations. It scares me to death that I have no control over achieving my unattainable goals. More frightening is that I honestly expected to fulfill the high ideals. Perhaps perfectionism is as addictive as the eating disorder. I search for the mistakes or shortcomings in my life, when all the while I am really doing okay.

"Maybe if I eat perfectly, eat less, and lose weight I will be closer to the right track." In reality there is no correlation between my weight or body and the status of my life. I use to envision this mystical world where within the loss of fat and weight lies paradise: decisions become easier, opportunities are in abundance, boys frolic all around, and clothes are a joy to try on, for they always look perfect. I was so sure that at 110 I would be in paradise or this paradise was awaiting me in this aerobics class. No, I know it is at 105. Actually I could have bet my life that somewhere in the next thirty pounds I would find it (peace). What I am finding is a big hole where I have stuffed this obsession for an eternally euphoric life in which my family, friends, and I would live happily ever after. The reality is that that's nothing more than a fantasy.

Maybe my fantasy is one way I have coped. All the pressure I placed on myself was a way to avoid the deeper vibration of truth. The food served as the catalyst that continually perpetuated the belief that I was in charge. I could drive myself as fast and as far as needed. Ultimately my food put a million miles of distraction between reality and me.

CO꒖CD

About ten girls from the ranch got to go to this Mexican food place called Anita's, then bowling. I had an assignment to eat a half of a quesadilla. I did fine, but some of the girls just lost it and started crying. The nurses had to go into the bathroom with the girls and talk them through their fears.

The people in the restaurant must think we are a bunch of freaks, crying over a tortilla chip and all. The poor waitress. I can just see them paying each other off to wait on the table of Remuda Ranch girls. Poor lady, she has no idea as she sets the plate down whether this one or the next one will burst into tears.

I really had fun tonight and I enjoyed being with myself for the first time in a while. The only real problem was waiting for the food. I became anxious. I also find myself obsessing over what is and what is not normal.

CO꒖CD

I feel so angry, like I am suffocating. In Body Image class we had to draw an outline of the way we saw our bodies and then our partners had to trace the real outlines of our bodies. I was so much skinnier than I thought. The therapist pointed out that I had drawn my breast but not my feet. She asked me why. The answer was simple. I have always loved that I have big boobs. I had not even acknowledged the fact that they no longer existed. I had wanted them there, so I imagined them into being. They are not even there anymore. I had just imagined that they were. It's like my thinking that I had put on a lot of weight, even though I still look really emaciated. Everything outlined before me I created in my mind and as painfully real as the drawing was, it had manifested itself into my outside world. I just couldn't get out of that classroom fast enough. I love my body. I used to love my body even before I got sick. The outline is the painful truth.

I cannot begin to recall in the month I have been here all the subtle ways God has helped my recovery progress. However, tonight God is not about subtleties. There is this young girl, about sixteen, four-feet nine and I am guessing sixty pounds. She was considered one of the old-timers. (That is my way of saying she had been there for more than two months). She said something to me that won't leave my mind. As always, before a meal we all stand in a in a circle to pray. A few of us were waiting on the other girls to answer the dinner bell. The young girl heard me talking about the body outline and that I found it very upsetting. She looked me straight in the face and said, "From the moment you got here you have thought that you were different from us. You're not. You are just like each one of us. You're an addict. Your story may differ, but you are emaciated, worn out, sick, and you are an addict. So don't think you are special or any different. When you accept where your life has taken you, only then will you start to grow, change, and begin to understand the word recovery."

∞∞

I began to understand from the moment I signed myself in into Remuda that no one made me have this disease, no single person had the power in my life to fuel my slow suicide. Now the truth is glaringly obvious: I chose it. As Dr. Don Durham would say, "I lit the match." Unfortunately there is not one cause, one reason, and it's not simply a bad habit. If that were true, I would have left weeks ago cured. There are many "logs on the fire," some put there by me, parents, experiences, and life. It is up to me now to take my life in a new direction, take charge of my tapestry, stop waiting for life to become perfect. Most of all I must admit that I am powerless over my addiction. I find myself terrified that Mom and Bill are here today, maybe because they are coming expecting the blame or thinking that once I leave Remuda this issue will be behind us and we can move on with our lives in an orderly fashion. My fear is of personal authenticity and truth. Since we as a family have not spoken the truth nor discussed the reality of our lives for the past few years, we have much to tell and much to learn. We must all have been terribly afraid. I know my parents thought they were doing the best thing by not talking. That is how shame, secrets, and denial grow. They grew within the darkness of the silence. Now it is up to me to take charge and tell the truth. My addiction is filled with lies and deception, and to bring that into the light seems unbearable. I have turned my Family Week over to God because I will only make a mess of it trying to make it just right.

LATER

I have had an array of emotions since they got here. Only half the troop has arrived. I feel indescribably strong. Being around them makes me realize how far I have come. I have experienced things they will never understand. I have felt things I may never share. As I look at them I see them searching for the girl they put on the plane a month ago. Still they look at me in hope of change, and perhaps even for a reason to hope. I never noticed the pain that must have been there all this time— so much sadness and despair. I want them to know what they do not know. Only time will reveal that I am changed. My changing is slow in coming, but these infinitesimal increments will be lasting. I am committed to life, to seeing into the life of things. I'm grateful for another day and that I will never live in that hell again. Most of all, God and I have taken charge. In my heart I know I finally belong.

Seeing them I am reminded of who and what I had become to the family—this moving body with little emotion, no expressions, or joy, just existing numbly, doing everything to nurture my addiction and feed the fire.

I still look forward to the next meal with excitement, which scares me. I don't like thinking and obsessing about food. There is so much more. I like food but not enough to have my life be about that. For the first time in two years I have the privilege of thoughts other than food.

When I went to the Family Week orientation tonight, Dad did the coolest thing. I love Easter and especially the bunny rabbits. On the phone last week I had asked him to send me a stuffed rabbit. He asked me to come outside and open his car. The entire inside was covered in stuffed bunny rabbits hung and placed all over the car. I was so excited. I just love Easter.

The Family Week began with the owners and founders of the ranch, Mr. and Mrs. Ward Keller. Mr. Keller talked about his story and why their family believed in starting Remuda. As I sat there and listened with five other families, I just started to cry. I could feel the intensity in every person and I was scared to death. I began to feel better. I just can't believe how blessed I am. I really feel like the luckiest girl in the world to have a family that loves me so much that they would come all this way. Mr. Keller asked us to set individual goals for this week. Mine is to trust God's plan and live in the moment! It pretty much sums up what I have been working on—well, at least one aspect.

Our Truth in Love is Tuesday. That is when I tell my family and the others all my secrets, admit stuff, and make amends for things. I also tell each person in my family what they did that hurt me. Then I will address my commitment to recovery as well as the steps I will take to stay in recovery. I think I might suffocate. Oh yes. They do the same, minus the secrets and my plan for recovery. I just want to let go of this week. I can't even imagine what it will be like. The thought of telling them all my secrets, and of rituals I have performed the past two-and-half-years makes me nauseous. Then I'll be telling them how they have pissed me off and talking about all the family secrets—I think I might die!

The support and love from my family is unbelievable. Tomorrow is the day when it all comes out. I told all of them when they got their sheets to fill out for the Truth in Love, where they will write out the amends and wounds, to not hold back because I was going full force and telling all. In other words don't let me get away with anything, because I was going to lay into them. I really believe that this is a critical part of my recovery.

I realized tonight that I am standing on my own, not with my family nor behind them but away and on my own. I feel like this is a battle of love versus this disease. The secrets keep me sick and I want no part of them. It will take true love to face this stuff honestly, but I believe in my family.

I am so exhausted I can hardly think. The Truth in Love went from 1:30 till 5:30. When we started I suddenly felt a great distance between us, as if at that moment we were all separate entities. It was the best and hardest thing I have ever done. Telling them how self-centered and absorbed I was in my addiction was awful (as if they didn't know) and then to tell them that I threw up when I said I wasn't and how I wanted them to hurt and I wanted to punish them by making them watch me starve. I told them I wanted attention and admitted that I really had no self-control and that I didn't care whether I lived or died, which was the bottom line. I was so humiliated. Whatever facade I tried to put up was gone now. Next was one thing I never thought I would explicitly describe. I openly talked about my being sexually abused (in a room full of relative strangers) first by Michael and then by Trisha, and it almost killed me. The shame became more intense with each word. I thought I would shatter my heart, the pounding was so strong. Thirty people all looked at me as I continued, wanting my knowledge out in the open. I willfully revealed the two most shaming and terrifying memories a child can have. My daily prayer that everyone would forget, I no longer needed. My deepest shame was now known by everyone. Secrets should never become prayers.

One of the deepest wounds I had was from my mom, because as far as I knew, nothing had ever been done about the abuse. I had never talked about that day. Therefore I kept the second time a secret for fourteen years. I asked her whether it made her mad. When she said, "Yes, it hurt more than anything" I got more upset. All this time I thought that because she did not respond, it was my fault. So I asked her to yell at Michael and tell him she hated him. She did, in a tearful voice, but I wanted to hear her scream at the top of her lungs "I HATE YOU MICHAEL!" (Never in all my life had she ever raised her voice, but something deep inside her gave her a raging strength.) John Holt just lost it, he was crying so hard. He knew it had happened, but no one had talked about it. I think hearing Mom scream what he had probably felt all those years freed him of a lot. The doctors had told my mom to hope, since I was only four, that I would forget. I think Bill and Dad were blown away by Mom's strength. I loved hearing her yell at that sick son of a bitch. I also felt it was really sad that she had all that inside for so long and never knew how much we all needed to know that she was hurting and that she could feel so angry. I swear you would have thought Michael in Texas had heard her. In her scream all I heard was, "Chelsea, you are my baby girl and never could it be your fault."

Then came my dad. He has always wanted for one of his children to go to Vanderbilt, and I was the last of a dying breed. I didn't want to go. When I told him, he had to take it well considering the surroundings, but he was crushed. Then I confronted him about the affair and how he left us and never paid child support and, from my perspective, lived the high life in L.A. while Mom struggled to make things work for us here. My dad was full of empty promises, which was a blessing and a curse. I never expected anything so I never really got hurt, but at the same time I never allowed myself to be vulnerable or accept his inconsistent love. He cleared stuff up and told me his side of the story, and although he had made mistakes, I found that my imagination had exaggerated them. But the truth is that I had grown up not knowing this man but had called him Dad.

He complained of his fear of being left out and of being just an intimidating person who writes checks but who is not involved in making decisions in my life. I wanted to say, "You were the one who chose to leave, and if our relationship has come to that I guess you should have thought things through before you made a lot of decisions." I am always amazed at his ability to blame me for the lack of cohesion between us. He claimed it was mostly my fault for not being available, for not calling or writing. It must get confusing trying to understand that he is the father and I am the child. He forgot more birthdays than he remembered, but I was starting to accept that that is the way he is, like it or not.

His wounds did not surprise me. I have always known how much it hurt him that we never spent time together. There were several years he reminded me of that I refused to see him. I sat and listened to him and my stepmother talk about how much I hurt them. It especially hurt them when I told them at the age of nine, "It hurts too much to love someone so much who lives far away." I was amazed that the rest of our conversation was not recalled by either of them because for me it was the most important part of the conversation: At nine I knew that something wasn't right with my dad. It wasn't that I didn't understand their divorce or that he never visited and rarely wrote. It wasn't that each time I visited I was introduced to a new girlfriend. There was something I didn't get but that I hated. I hated how he and Jude yelled so loudly at each other and fought like beasts. I remember at the time telling myself it wasn't my dad but maybe Jude or maybe his drinking. It has taken me along time to realize that he poured the drink in his hand and that he was far from a victim of circumstance. Bottom line—I was afraid of being with my dad. There was so much unpredictable behavior going on it seemed unwise to depend on him at all. I wanted no part of that scary place he called home.

There was no sense in clouding the air with accusations. I knew what he and I both wanted was to be heard, so to the best of my ability I listened. I saw pain in his eyes and for the first time caught a glimpse of the dad I had always imagined he would have been had he raised me. Thank you, God, because I have found hope in our relationship. Seeing his life through his eyes was something that never dawned on me, but as he spoke the truth in his heart I began to see. I know in my silence he must have heard how much I needed and wanted to be Dad's little girl. I dove into his arms. I wished that moment would never end. He said something I had heard him say before but not until now had it made sense. "There is nothing more powerful than truth. The truth is something you can not add to or take away from: It is simply the truth."

Truth is the only thing that could come close to describing today. My secrets had been an unbridgeable gulf between us. Something as simple as breathing the truth into our lives began to repair all we had known our family to be. My family, bless them, they did not force feed me, berate me, or send me to my room. They waited—waited for me to turn back to them on my own, back to life. Their willingness to risk vulnerability, to express themselves authentically, allowed them to change in their own right. Today was the highest reflection of our souls. Today was the first day I began to truly love my father. Truth is amazing—amazingly giving. All this and a deeper knowledge of who resides within the sanctuary of my heart. There would never be another day like it in my life—I wanted time to stand still.

∞∞∞

Where do I begin? My eyes are still almost swollen shut. I am in shock over yesterday and how powerful every moment was. Never could I have dreamed of such an epiphany of healing for the whole family. It almost killed my mother. She has been holding on to a lot of stuff for a long time. I really had no idea the extent to which my family was affected by my eating disorder. Hearing its impact was so important. God, thank you so much for yesterday. I truly believe that not until I sat before my family was I strong enough. When the time came, you made me strong enough to live the truth. I am so blessed by such an incredible family.

Dr. Don said that my eating disorder was a way for me to relieve myself from the role and the pressure of being the perfect kid, the one who carried all the family tension and responsibility. My disease was a harsh way of physically expressing my emotional turmoil.

I am so tired of using food to make me happy. I think about my next meal and what it will be. I hate being obsessed with it. I am not about food anymore. It is still a way for me to escape from my feelings. But this idea that the next meal or the shape of my body will make me happy is not true. I have been fooling myself by thinking I can do it my way and I can just eat like a normal person when I get home. I need my meal plan, and I need to follow my recovery plan to a T. The groups, counseling, church, and journaling are all vital to my success, and I will be damned if I will waste any more of my life on this.

I am not healed and I need to realize that I am always one choice away from my addiction. I don't know why I feel so lonely right now. I am really exhausted. I have been feeling and thinking so much that I just need to sit and do nothing, maybe watch TV. Sometimes I wish that this would all be over.

Without recovery being my number one priority, I have no life and I will die, maybe not from starvation but by killing the person I am growing up to be. I love Helen Keller's idea: "Life is either a daring adventure or nothing at all." I need to acquire a taste and craving for adventure and not always search for security. My time at Remuda cannot be spent getting rid of this disease or simply learning to move on with my life. It must be spent realizing life is not about security but adventure and taking whatever the day holds. I really believe that my adventure will never get off the ground without my acceptance of full responsibility for my life and my recovery. I must want it and be ready to fight like hell to keep it. I will, with God's help.

Last night was GREAT! Mom, Dad, John Holt, and I went to Sun City, Phoenix, for dinner at Sfuzzi's. It was so good. I had an assignment to have Dad order my dinner for me.

Amy, my therapist, did this to challenge my willingness to let go
and not be so controlling over my food. Well, it proved to be a
challenge to say the least. First, Dad ordered fried calamari.
Next he ordered roasted chicken and vegetables marinated in
olive oil. I didn't think he would order that. Sitting there hearing my meal ordered for me was torture. Tears filled my eyes. I
was so scared and felt that my feelings didn't matter and that I
just had to eat it. In all honesty I didn't like how fattening my
meal was going to be, nor did I like not having control over
what was going to go in my body. I was taken with what a big
deal I made one meal out to be. The three minutes of ordering
became my life's destiny.

When the waiter left, as a family we did something different. We talked about my fear. I began to realize that this was
just a meal—great food—and in the "grand scheme of my eating plan," it would have no effect. Talking about it was just
what I needed. The lump in my throat was dissolving. I knew I
could do it. Right then we prayed together as a family for God
to be present and for God to give me courage. The meal continued. I took a lot of deep breaths. Even though it didn't feel
right, I knew the action was right. I acted as if it felt perfectly
normal. I continued eating, trusting that my actions were good
but knowing that I would not enjoy a meal for some time.
Ultimately the feelings would come to pass, once I got out of
my head and lived the reality that I was okay. We laughed forever at John Holt's amazing humor and Dad's quick wit. We
finished with a flourless chocolate cake and cappuccino. We
laughed and laughed. I couldn't help but think how much
laughter I must have missed. I experienced life last night, and I
am in love with it. I was so happy, I am so happy. I can actually say that I am grateful for the hard times I've had and the ones
I have not yet come to know. In return, I felt life last night.

I hated returning to the ranch because all the patients had

a virus. I will die if I get it. Mom and I have planned to go shopping in Phoenix today. First we will meet Dad and J.H. for breakfast before they go back. I am nervous about shopping because I have gained weight and it will be hard.

∞∞

The morning routine has become almost humorous when I think what my friends would say if they were watching. Grey and I wake up at 6:00 or 6:30 to the alarm. Grey begins to read her Bible. I pray and read a few verses myself. Then, on alternating days, put on the paper robe and walk in the dark to the main lodge. I am greeted by many half-asleep women waiting in line to step on the scale. I turn my back to the scale while the nurse reads and records my weight. The numbers are not discussed until you reach a certain level of progress. Then knowing the number becomes optional. I do not want to know my weight, mostly because of the mind game, the control I would give a dumb number over my life, self-esteem, and mental well-being. Even if the scale reads less than my assumption, the verdict would still dictate my happiness. I run back down the lighted path because it is pretty cold. The stars are so amazing here, still brilliantly aglow. I get dressed for the day. I take time to put lotion on. They say that is important because we need to nurture our bodies. My clothes are more snug than when I came, but to my surprise I am proud. Grey and I return to the main lodge for breakfast, which is always served in the dining area. I find my place card, get my water, and meet the rest in a circle to pray before we sit and eat breakfast. Then my favorite part of the day, chapel. I just love all the songs we sing. Both of the visiting ministers are so great and give sermons that really apply well to our lives and present situation. Depending on the day and what group you are in your schedule of activities is determined. Some patients go to Equine for the morning, a class called Relapse Prevention, group, or individual therapy. A bell around 12:30 brings us all back together for lunch. The afternoon activities might be nutrition (with the nutritionist), Body Image, or art therapy, and then we all meet together for didactic with Dr. Don Durham. The topic is different each day but always fun and interesting.

꩜

I had an ice cream cone today! I hate that I always seem to eat more than my meal plan. I am just so excited to be eating. Monica, the nutritionist, takes all these figures and measurements to establish our individual weight range. Then she gives us a meal plan that we are to earnestly follow. For example, lunch will be two meats, three breads, one fat, one fruit, and one vegetable. I think the whole meal plan is a big relief. I don't know how or what to eat, and this way I have been told. I just follow the rules. Following the plan is hard. For so long I have not allowed myself a whole slice of bread. Anyway back to the ice cream. I loved every bite, and I am still here to talk about it.

I had to talk to my parents about how terrified I am of coming home, back to the world where I was so sick. Even though I have changed, the context of my surroundings at home will not have changed. Reentering real life is so frightening. Everyone will know that I was at a treatment center. I can't hide the fact that I have an eating disorder and that now I am a person in recovery from an eating disorder. Facing my friends, their parents, and even the people I don't know who are familiar with a very private chapter of my life will not be easy. I left behind many secrets that are not only public knowledge but probably fabricated by now.

It's funny my mind told me eating ice cream would make me fat, then that feeling becomes a fact in my mind, that I really have become fat. They (Remuda) say that fat is not a feeling.

As I began to talk about my fear of leaving Remuda, I realized my feelings had nothing to do with ice cream or fat. My fear of returning and facing the unknown was eating me up inside. Knowing that food cannot cause fear nor can it fix my fears is a relief. Even though I feel alone and frightened, all I have to do is today and I can handle that.

I am not leaving Remuda fixed, but I am leaving with the knowledge and understanding that I will be discovering for the rest of my life who I am and where I am going, one day at a time. I am not my body, numbers, appearance, size, my disease, or perfect. These things are only character traits. They are mere shadows of the best parts of me, the parts I love the most. These shadows no longer define me. My health has no room for those who see me for my disease and symptoms.

For my family, I praise you Lord. They are everything I need. Completely supportive, loving, honest, caring, and truthful. They dropped everything to experience healing with me and fight this battle with me. I could never trade a moment for what I had with them during Family Week. When Mom, Dad, and John Holt came back and I witnessed my parents tell each other they do love one another despite all that has happened. Seeing them forgive one another was the greatest gift, because I had no other choice but to forgive. My mom is very loving to tell my dad his mistakes were merely that, just mistakes. I don't know how she could have been so forgiving, because I think having an affair is the worst thing. As a result of his choice, he sacrificed being a father, raising us, and fulfilling his responsibilities. He helped raise John Holt and Ashley during their younger years. Without sounding resentful, he was more biology than a father to me. I hope he realizes how badly he screwed up. I never bought his excuse that Fort Worth wasn't right for him. If he did not like Fort Worth all he needed to do was say so. I know we would have all moved in a heartbeat. Instead, he left and started a new life, leaving behind the day-to-day responsibilities of being a father. I am eighteen years old. He has never seen me off to school, met one of my dates, poured my cereal, or even punished me for being out to late. Ashley and John Holt know him differently than I. I know they have a different perspective of him as a father.

☞☜

I am not in a good place. Dad told me that I did not get accepted to Vanderbilt. You would think I would be relieved, but I hate the fact that they told me no. Basically, Vanderbilt is saying that I am not good enough to go there. I worked so hard all through school so I could have choices about where I would go to college. I am horrible at standardized tests. I thought Vanderbilt would look at more than just my SAT score. After eating a healthy breakfast I became very antsy. The news was driving me crazy. I just feel so dumb. The urge was so strong to go and binge. I really feel like a failure and bad about myself because I wasn't good enough for them. Now this means that I go to University of Texas summer school and see if I can make it through the provisional program to be admitted for the fall. It really scares me that I would even consider throwing up, or even worse, crave it. I can't handle this on my own. When I went shopping I got clothes, but then got upset because I didn't feel like I deserved them. I think about food all the time, but when I am down on myself. It feels like I am doing it all wrong. Recovery seems impossible. I continue to believe that obsessing about food will take away my feelings of inadequacy. Maybe I just don't know where else to turn. Maybe I need to teach myself a healthier way of thinking. I have chosen the lies to lead my thoughts. I must choose not to believe the bad. My mind sorts my thoughts into extremes. Something is either good or bad, disgusting or beautiful. This black-and-white thinking is purely destructive.

I did it; I am home in my bed! I could hardly contain myself tonight. When I got off the airplane all my friends were waiting for me. I dropped my bags and took off in a dead sprint. I leaped into their arms. We couldn't stop screaming and crying. Lauren looked me straight in the eyes and with tears running down her cheeks said, "I have my Chelsea back. Your eyes are alive and I was so afraid I would never see them shine again." We talked and laughed forever. I never realized how much I was missing in my life. I never knew how afraid all of my friends were of losing me. I was so sick I had no concept of enjoying life, much less my life as a seventeen-year-old. I was so proud of my success, I wanted them to see how much I had changed and they did. I was really excited for them to see me eat. I had been craving Taco Bueno. All they could say was how grateful they were to have me back and healthy. I couldn't wait to tell them all about Remuda.

The first thing I needed to do was to explicitly tell them about my triggers, the signs to watch for, and most of all to ask, not assume or be afraid to tell me they are concerned. Everyone is involved in my recovery. Recovery is part of me and I want them involved in my life. The secrecy keeps me sick. My symptoms must become a matter of fact not a matter of fault. It feels so good to need and want people. It seems to come as a surprise that recovery is a process and that I am not "fixed." I explained to them that I, unlike others, believe with all my heart that someday I will be in a very different place with my recovery as well as my issues with food. In other words, I will not always struggle in my recovery and with food. When I do, I know it is a red flag that there is something much more going on than just food, and I need to be open to what lies in front of me. It is almost like my body is speaking a different language. My mind will say, "Your thighs are getting bigger, your stomach is so flabby, your pants are tighter than they were yesterday. You should not have eaten all the sandwich. Now you are going to gain weight. I know that cookie was more than you should have had and now you are going to get fat." Oh, and one of my favorites, "You really have put on a few pounds, you better not . . . or else you are going to really get fat and gross." Instead of listening to these lies, I need to ask, "What is the truth," remind myself "fat is not a feeling," and also look at what has been going on in my life that might have triggered these thoughts. I really hope they understood. If they don't, I can't blame them because I myself have trouble understanding most of the time. Eating disorders are baffling, especially for those who have never had negative thoughts or feelings about food and their bodies. I don't always understand why I chose my body as an outlet for my feelings and emotions.

Tomorrow I am going to Mimi's for her famous breakfast. She and Pampaw were so sweet while I was at Remuda. They wrote me all the time. I know this whole deal was really hard on them and difficult to understand. I can't say I was surprised that when Mom talked to them about the abuse they denied it happened. They felt that I probably childishly fabricated the events and it wasn't as serious as everyone was making it out to be. I had hoped the truth of the abuse would help them understand partly why I was destroying my body. I don't blame them for denying or minimizing what happened. I wouldn't want anything like that for any child, much less my own grandchild. I just hope when they see me, the abuse is not all they see or all they think about.

This eating is all pretty scary. I am eating really normally and I keep hearing these "what ifs." I just have no idea what to expect for the next few months of my life. I want to start seeing the best in people. I am making that a goal for myself. If I look for the best in others, then I believe I will look for the best in myself.

Getting excited about a day at Remuda was easy. I lived in a little bubble where we were all so protected. We focused on ourselves and recovery. I always knew no matter the pain or the feeling, somehow it would come out and be addressed, ultimately evoking good out of pain. Never before had I been so close to God. I really knew he was watching over me and protecting me.

My body image has been really negative lately. Sitting still is so hard. When I sit still I have to think about the stuff going on inside my head and deal with it. What if I don't do this right (recovery)? What if I don't say and do the things I should? Will I be punished, will I end up an emaciated woman for the rest of my life? If I am alone or if God abandons me I might die. I can't do this alone.

I think a lot about a woman named Sally. She came to Remuda about two weeks after I did. Well into a month of her treatment she lost it during lunch. I knew Sally was really struggling with her addiction to exercise, but when she refused to eat her grilled cheese, I knew her objection was just the tip of her pain. After the assigned table nurse calmly asked her to eat the sandwich I couldn't help but notice the table was vibrating profusely. My eyes switched to Sally's knees bouncing up and down, as though she was running a seated marathon. The longer she resisted and refused to talk, the faster her legs moved. Tears were running down her face. One look around the room and the domino effect was obvious. Every woman and girl had stopped eating, inconspicuously pushed her plate away, or drifted to another place. Now don't get me wrong. I really liked Sally, but something had to be done. I knew if I came to her rescue in any consoling way, I would hear about it in group. What felt like an eternity before the nurse finally interjected was no more than a few seconds. Sally slowly began to talk. Of all days for me to be seated next to her, why on the day of great confession? Hanging her head as low as possible she began to speak softly, "I've been sneaking off after meals and throwing up. I have been exercising by doing sit-ups and push-ups in my room." The next thing I knew, Sally bolted from the table and several nurses went after her. Girls were all upset and crying. The whole scene was awful. That day was one of the few times I ever lost my cool during a meal. I started crying and despite my grave efforts to gain control, the "cool and collected" patient was terrified and cried in fear.

After lunch I found Kay Ward, the owner of Remuda. Of course she had already heard of the outbreak, but I wanted help in understanding why Sally's failure in recovery upset me and why her resistance mattered. Why had her not eating and lying terrified me so? Kay did what I needed most—she listened. Her silence allowed me to understand my fear on my own. Her loving, motherly eyes encouraged every word I hesitated to release. The reality was that Sally's slip was my greatest fear. Fear of the pain that made her choose to lie and abuse her body, her apparent desperation and shame, I couldn't bear to feel again. I wanted Kay to give me the answer, I wanted her to give me the key. I wanted to know what would keep me from failing like Sally. What would make my recovery last? Kay's beautiful smile encouraged my anticipation of the secret she was about to unveil. "Chelsea, I don't know. That is for you to find for yourself." I cried harder because I hadn't a clue. I've thought about our conversation several times a day since we talked. She was right. I need to discover the answer each day for myself.

I realized a lot that day. In many ways Remuda changed forever in my eyes. I began to see patients as a mirrors, some reflecting what I don't want to be and some whom I hope to reflect. Each patient in her unique stage of recovery showed me the lies and the truth, that I am just like Sally and I can make the same choices. This process will take time and I will feel that pain again. Mirrors had always been painful, but that day I learned that I could look to them and find a precious gift. The reality that the old way is waiting to embrace me with open arms, the truth that I really am one move, one choice away from hell and sheer pain, frightens and scares me shitless. I am crying right now over the uncertainty of my success in recovery. I just never want to be in so much pain or hate myself enough to do that again, to live like that again. I have learned that I am so much more and that I don't have to. I can be blind to my choices and get caught in the momentum of the rituals, hearing that voice that takes over. The mutiny in my mind is the worst suffocation imaginable. With everything in me I don't want to be her again, but wanting is not enough. I wish there was security in the unknown.

When I stick my fingers down my throat, it's as if I can reach the nasty feeling, the darkness, all the disgusting stuff inside me and all that my mind tells me. My hand carries out some of the crap and darkness that fills the inside of me. For a moment my darkness is still, like there is nothing else wrong in my world and that stuff inside that is so dark stops for just a moment. I can live with myself. I can accept me, that which I believe no one else can. In that moment I know peace. I really believe that somehow my hand can pull out those horrible feelings of worthlessness and almost punish them for being there. I am so angry, but it won't go away. Inside it is just so fucking dark and disgusting. My actions feel so appropriate to the pain I am feeling. I just can't breathe, I just want to breathe. I know that my heart is red and is filled with good stuff, but it is submerged in this hell that makes up the rest of my body. It doesn't take but a second to realize that my attempt was unsuccessful, but it tells me I can carry on. At least my efforts make the outside look different from the way I feel on the inside. I guess when you feel so fucking bad about yourself and so help-less over those feelings, they became uncontrollable. I feel so worthless that for me the physical pain of throwing up and the pain I inflict on my throat seems an appropriate punishment for the crap that consumes me. It is no different when I starve. I can just punish myself for feeling like that. I turn inside by starving those feelings away and by shutting down. I tell myself, I don't deserve to eat. If I can't get myself right, how can I get anything right in my life? Once again I affirm my feel-ings of worthlessness.

They told me that I was expecting too much out of my recovery and that I would throw up again. When I do throw up again I need to talk about my feelings and admit that I did throw up. Most important, pick up where I left off and EAT THE NEXT MEAL. Oh, I am always supposed to try to delay for at least forty-five minutes and hope the urge will pass. I call someone on my support list of friends and talk. The same goes for restricting and deviating from Remuda's eating regimen. I must be open and talk to someone even when I swear it is just that I don't want to eat because I am getting fat or I am "just not hungry." I am determined not to throw up ever again. For some reason my saying that really seemed to scare my coun-selors at Remuda.

∞∞

Yesterday was really hard. I was completely obsessed about my body. It took me quite awhile to realize what was really going on and the reality that there was something other than my size bothering me. The control and comfort of my addic-tion has been removed. I am struggling to find a way to live without it. When I imagine going to college in Austin in a few months, it terrifies me. I just arrived home from Remuda and now I have to leave again. All I can do is today. I am not ready for Austin or I would be there. I am going to my support group tonight. This is a new ritual for me. My ritual is three meetings a week, meet with my therapist, Cheryl, once a week, and go to church. Sometimes I don't want to, but I just do because it is where my life is right now and it is a major part of recovery. As Dr. Don would say, "You do it because it is a new ritual. It doesn't matter if you feel like it or not. You do it because it is a new behavior."

∞∞

I thought I would never be able to walk down the halls at school now that everyone knows my big secret. Being honest about going to Remuda was the best choice. Everyone, I mean everyone, even the janitor, told me he was proud of me. Teachers and students I hardly know have told me they are glad to see me back and are so relieved that I am healthy again. I was forewarned of the compliments people would make when I returned. A tough one is, "You look so healthy." Now to the average person that is a fine compliment. To an eating disordered person "healthy" equals "fat." I remind myself that is not what they mean. I also cringe when a person deems it necessary to reiterate how horrible I looked, how disgusting I was, how gross my bony shoulders were, and that they are just so, so glad that I have a full face now and my jeans are tight. I have become good at realizing they are just as fearful of my relapse as I am. My appearance is better, but I wish they knew that I am not proud of the way I treated my body and the way I made it look.

I must say I have had some wonderful compliments, some of which I really take to heart. My favorite was from Kevin. Kevin and I became great friends my freshman year. He came to my rescue when some other guys were playfully teasing me. Kevin's six-foot-five, 250-pound, pure muscle build I always found comforting in any situation. His being black is irrelevant other than for the sake of my understanding the cultural context of his compliment. I saw him towering over every head in the hall and his strong voice came down the hall saying, "Mmmm, Chelsea! you are lookin' sooo gooood. You know what I love most? Do you know what I love most?" I smiled because I knew what was coming next and there wasn't a damn thing I could do about it as he continued, "You got your big bootie back." He continued toward me singing, "Chelsea 'got back' Chelsea 'got back' (paying homage to his favorite song "Baby Got Back"). He scooped me up in his arms and said, "I am so glad to see the Chelsea I fell in love with." Having an apple butt in Kevin's eyes was the greatest of all attributes. After that I realized all compliments must be understood through their eyes, not mine.

I had the best time at this party. I danced forever. I swear dancing is one of my favorite things. I feel so free and have so much fun. I love to do crazy moves and make Lauren and Elizabeth laugh. I love spending time with them. They have been so supportive. I know it is not easy for them to ask how my recovery is going, but I feel relieved when they do. It is on all our minds, and I want to be honest with them and share my life with them. I want them in my life.

It must be normal to feel that you lose your way and who you are at times. Maybe that's how I learn who I am. Through experiencing the uncertainty, I become more sure of the stuff that makes me Chelsea. The shadows are proving as valuable as the light. I can take the stuff I want and leave the things I don't. I can never lose sight of the fact that I must love and believe in myself.

Learning to let others love me by loving myself has always been true.

☙☙

The days are passing, and it saddens me. Graduation is so close.

∞∞

Consider the source; I was bombarded by David with comparisons about my body and my neck being too big. I have been struggling since then with being too heavy. I am scared. My eyes will always confirm what my mind tells them is there. Accepting change is letting go. Letting go enough to trust that God is putting me in a better place. I know this to be true for other aspects of my life, like my relationships and school, so it must be true for my body as well. I doubt God is sitting up in heaven saying, "Chelsea your time to change has come. I want your neck to be big and your waist to grow two inches." I do think that my body changing is part of its natural course and somehow mixes in with God's plan. I do believe he cares because he knows how much I do. Also I would so much rather be like I am now, healthier, stronger, and full of life. Writing my thoughts about God or my new ways of thinking and new lingo makes it all the more real for me. I don't want to forget the healthy stuff. I know I will need it. God, please protect me and put to rest my fear that you will not take care of my weight and appearance. Nothing you give me can I not handle. Word for the day: Responsibility.

∞∞

One of the recommendations from Remuda is to find a good dietitian. Well, I went to this female dietitian who was suppose to be great. Now I am all worked up. Granted she has the worst job in the world, dealing with eating-disordered neurotics all day, myself included. However, she should know when I ask her if fries or desserts are okay once or twice a week, not to look at me with these gaping eyes and say, "Well not if you want to stay the way you are now. Mind you are on a mainte-nance diet." I was hoping she would give me this big pat on the back for voluntarily eating such "sin." I couldn't tell you what the blubbering idiot said after that. My mind was mapping out the course of my four-mile run that would start at the appoint-ment's close.

I have allowed her to get in my head. I am afraid to eat any of my fattier meat choices, like peanut butter, or red meat, where I wasn't before. I mean I am not going to eat all the fries and pie that cross my plate, but she did not need to scare me with all the weight that might happen if I don't do it right. Not doing anything just right scares me to death, much less my food intake. Dumb lady, I won't see her again. I decided it wasn't worth my recovery to freak out and go run. I sat here and wrote to you, God, instead.

Something else must be going on for her to have upset me so. God, please help me look inside and not buy into the feel-ing that food is my problem. Help me let go of the food issue. I hate worrying about it. I have been talking to another girl about her eating disorder. I told her that she can be as skinny as she wants and no one can stop her. I had to tell her when she asked me point blank how I lost all my weight that I wouldn't write her a prescription to kill herself. Sort of corny, but I was at a loss for words. I wanted to say, "Hell no I won't tell you. Are you crazy?" Who knows what the right thing to say is? It is a mystery to me and I lived it. Sometimes I think about how frustrating I must have been to my family. I have been right where this girl was, but I still wanted to shake some sense into her head.

∞∞

I got my period yesterday! After two years! I love you God. Thank you for restoring my body to be strong enough to do that. I feel so much joy right now, thank you. I struggled yesterday. I thought having my period made me fat, now I am grateful for the growth. I am excited. Please take my hand and lead me, because all I see is the inch in front of me. Word for the day: play.

⌒⌒⌒

This morning as I lie here in bed, fears of what I hate most rush through my head. Please, God, take them away, the pinching, feeling, and all the negative body image. I don't want to look like I did my freshman year when I was chubby. What if I lose all the muscle I built up? I know I eat sometimes because it tastes good or I am excited or anxious. Please help me be aware of those times and help me. God, I don't have control over this disease. Please, I beg you, take it over and put my heart and mind to rest. I hate this crap because I really love my body under all these lies: I need help not to turn my feelings inside today. I need to get my feelings out and stop accepting them as fact and holding them inside to hurt myself. I hate not being in control and not being patient with my friends and family. I go crazy when these thoughts take over, but I cannot change other people. Not eating or mentally ripping apart my body will not change others. I don't always have to be so strong. I am human.

I found myself trying to take care of everyone. I can tell how I really like to fix people. I do this by making myself extra good or extra special, to make their bad mood better. I defiantly don't want to be this person who rescues everyone.

The next twenty-four hours is all I have to do. God, please help me live today. I turn the control over to you. Hell, I don't know what I am or whether I am doing anything right anymore. I am trying to live a completely different life while still living in the same head with the same thoughts that got me into this obsession.

No one is going to bail me out if I relapse, nor can any-one replace that wasted time. I now accept the responsibility for how I live. This thought frightens me at first, but when I am more accepting of myself and others, I feel at peace, and I feel a sense of freedom. This can be a beautiful transition, and I should love it in its entirety. When I do experience sadness, I realize that it's not that the sadness has just come—it has been with me all along. But now I am aware of the sadness. I am ready to accept this feeling. Fate does not come to me from the outside in but from the inside out. I can remain standing and healthy in the midst of a transition. Word for the day: synthesis.

∽∽

Yesterday I learned that when I don't feel God's presence, I must keep walking as though he has always been with me and act as though he is. I really believe in Alanon and its role in my continuing in recovery. This woman came up to me after my meeting this evening and said that I was beautiful and that I was everything she wanted to be. Tears filled my eyes as she continued, "This is an appreciation not a compliment." My tears welled from many things. The fact that anyone could see beauty in me was so beyond any place I had been or way I had felt about myself. I really felt sadness over how I have never seen myself as she did and over the fact that a perfect stranger could be as honest as she was with me. I was grateful she took the time to tell me. She helped me realize the things I tell myself are so cruel and so unimportant in the heart of life. Accepting her appreciation has left me to struggle. But I will struggle well with this.

This committee meets in my head and not only creates chaos but also speaks to me as if I were some heinous person or some abusive demon who needs to be locked up. I am a healthy, loving person and I need to acknowledge those qualities.

Perhaps, I need to give myself a rest. Obviously I am like most people in that I don't see myself accurately.

When I lose God during the day I am trying to take control. I stop trusting that God is always there and that he is taking care of me. It happens when I stop letting go and resist. I become afraid and I fall. My body is changing. It is so easy to focus on the physical change and not all the positive things in my recovery. Word for the day: adventure.

꩜

Today, I wanted to throw up more than I have in a long time. I wanted to run. I wanted to run so far and so fast that the thoughts would not find me—I wanted to escape myself. I took a bath. I sit here knowing I resisted what seemed an unbearable urge. I have not thrown up since I began at Remuda. I am working hard. God is working. It is weird how I started to believe that I would never come out of that mood, that I could not escape without giving in to my desires and my urgency to fix things. But I did escape; I won. A definite downward spiral starts when things go bad. My mind allows every negative and bad thought to take control. It happens so fast. Even when I catch myself halfway into it, the thoughts don't want to let up. I hate that I love to beat myself up. I am afraid if I talk myself out of it I would be lying by not accepting those thoughts. The strange part is that I am lying. Those thoughts are lies. They grow stronger as I give in to them, as I spiral down. Jesus, I need you to help stop the spiral. I am proud and I feel joy right now. I am filled right now. Nothing else matters more than the moment I am living.

꩜

My spiral began the minute I woke up. I wanted to go run my ass off, literally. I really started to believe that I was fat. I could feel the excess. I tried to stop it, but it scared me to believe that my thoughts were lies. I didn't want to believe I was okay. If I believed I was okay and I wasn't, I would have a false confidence, and a faith in myself than I should not have. I mean, I would actually think I deserved to walk tall and proud even if I was a few pounds over. I don't have control over my weight anymore. I must trust God with whatever happens. Whatever happens, it will be another learning experience. I want to turn my fear over to God. I drowned in all those fears and they keep me from living in the moment. Today I want to live each moment, even if I need to take small steps to do so. I pray today for the courage to live with myself and to learn whatever the lessons are today. I will let go of my habit of being afraid and my assumed need to be afraid.

∞∞

I hate it. High school is coming to an end. I do not want to leave. I don't feel ready to take off and go to a totally new environment and leave all my support systems. I wore these shorts last night that fit, well, too tight. I have thought of every way to lose weight since I put the shorts on. I do not want to slowly creep to a size 8. I don't want to worry or think about this crap either. If I was a size 8 I am terrified of how ugly and fat I would be. What a lie. Damn it, what is going on in my head? I feel empty and afraid. All I have is today. But I am so lost, I can't do anything right. I feel so responsible for my family and my friends being happy, for their enjoyment of life. I feel like I have to make them enjoy me when I am around. I hate that I can't make everything good for them. I try so hard but I fail. Something happens to mess up a perfect situation. I'll say something dumb or ask the wrong question. I wish I could always do it right. I feel like they have this scoreboard where a constant tally of my screw-ups are documented. One day I am going to cross my line. I will have done so many wrong things that they will leave me without thinking twice about our relationship. If a friendship has tension, it is my fault. If a person is mad at me it is my fault. If there is silence, boredom, or sadness, the situation becomes my job to fix. In some way my eating disorder was a way to escape this self-imposed burden. I am scared to leave. Living in a new world in a new way scares me, because I don't know whether I will just go crazy and eat out of control, even though my life is so much healthier. I will focus on the joy in today.

Today will be everything it needs to be. I am powerless over my disease. I can make a choice to live today or die in it. I choose life with Jesus. God, please help me not try to control and manipulate people. Help me identify the times I do. Please give me your strength, Lord. Walk with me every minute and help me through the hard times in life. I can do it with your strength.

∞

A month ago I was freaked out about leaving for college . When I look how far I have come in my recovery, (especially in my willingness to go to Austin) I am shocked. It really is God's strength that has brought me here today. I pray for the trust and ability to let go and hand it over to you, God. How do I know that going to summer school in Austin will not be the best thing? Today is all I have. There is so much life to live today. I will write this on my heart. I feel awful in those lies, living out my lies. I am not about them. I am God's child. I pray for you to work and be in my life today. Please help me not doubt myself with those lies. That is not you or me. Word for today: abundance (what a great word).

∞

Obviously Bret knows that I am in recovery from an eating disorder, but I want to share more about it with him.

Talking about my struggles is a relief. The burden is released to some degree when I share my feelings and experience with Bret. I think I handled it well. I explained that I needed him to ask more about my disease/recovery and that in general I need to talk more about it. I have been holding back to protect him. I didn't want him to know that I wasn't just this perfect girl. I didn't think he wanted all this crap with a relationship. I am afraid my disease would be a bunch of junk to him. However, if we do not make it an open topic, I will remain just this weird screwed-up girl who wouldn't eat. I want him involved in my life.

Explaining to any male what, why, and how eating disorders are what they are is an arduous task. I try so hard to steer them free of the simplified stigma: "She doesn't eat, she wants to be skinny, and doesn't feel like she has control over her life." My not eating, purging, and being this way were symptoms, not the cause. My faulty perception and interpretation of my place in the world existed long before I waged my war with food. The problems had already taken root. I want him to have the chance to understand. I want to know he cares enough to try to understand. It scares me opening such a private part of myself and being vulnerable to his words, his response, or lack of response to what I share with him. What if we break up? What if he doesn't want to understand and he looks at me like some freak of nature who is gross and messed up? I am better off knowing where he stands now than later. Besides I can't deny where my life has led me. I can't go on not being honest.

∞∞

It was four months ago today that I entered treatment. Last night I drove for about an hour and half. I didn't solve anything. I just wanted to run, to just go. I turned the music up so loud, praying it would drown out the chaos and fear that consumed me. These changes are killing me. Without you, Lord, I know I couldn't do it. A few times the word "attention" crossed my mind. Run away, be in a wreck, and see how people would respond. I wanted attention, the same attention that I received from my eating disorder. The same kind of attention that ensured no one would be mad at me or blame me for anything. A true victim of circumstance. It kills me because I do and think so many things that are out of my sickness. I hate that. I don't want that. I thought my eating disorder was demanding. Recovery is ten times as hard..

∞∞

I chose not to write this morning. I didn't feel like it. I took some laxative tea last night. That was eating disorder behavior and I chose to do it. I think I will throw the stuff away. God, I am really scared. I think I need to tell Bret that I was sexually abused. I can still feel those shameful feelings. They don't belong, but they are there. I think I might feel more comfortable with him if he knows. My mind won't stay still when I am kissing him. It makes me sad that the abuse is still controlling me. I am going to tell him. That's all there is to it. Just suck it up. I think I might die I am so ashamed. I feel so bad and wrong for having this be part of my life. This is getting honest. This is really hard to say. God please help me.

∞∞

I can't believe this is my last day of high school. I don't want it to end. I don't want to go to college. I like my life fine, just the way it is. My conversation with Bret went so well. I couldn't believe how caring and understanding he was. He really didn't think I was weird, and he was also glad to hear that I wanted to talk more about my recovery. I can't help but feel closer to him since our talk. When I opened up to him, so much seemed to change for the better. He is so sweet. I know the relationship will end when I leave, but if I stay because of him, I would only end up resenting him. I am graduating today. I can't believe it.

# Secrets Revealed

B ill and I married four years after my divorce. We each
brought three children to the marriage. It was a blended
family that worked with lots of effort on every member's
part. One of the unifying forces was the baby of the family,
Chelsea. Chelsea was not more special or more binding than
the other children, but she was the most innocent, being only
one and a half when Bill and I started dating. She came into
our new family with less old baggage, fewer memories, fewer
scars, and more hope for the future, because she had less experience with the reality of the past. In the four years Bill and I
dated, and as our children began to take on their new roles in
our family, Chelsea carved out a place we were all thrilled for
her to take. She became the happy child, the loving one, the one
that could break tension between members of a step family, the
one who would hug whomever was hurting or feeling left out,
the one who could make the angry one laugh or the sad one
smile. All members of a step family have something to grieve,
but we thought she had less to grieve because she had no memory of a nuclear family with a biological father at Christmas or
birthdays. In reality she had more to grieve because she never
had those memories or experiences at all. Moreover, a year
before we married, Chelsea began to cover the undeserved

*shame of sexual assault. We did not know she felt this shame because she became a master at disguising fear. She became more skilled at playing the role she had assumed in the first three years we dated. However, the cost of being the perfect little girl was beginning to grow. Later it would compound, and the price was almost her life.*

*Chelsea at five and six seemed to have no cares, only caresses. She rarely misbehaved, and when she did, it usually made everyone chuckle. Of course she bugged her older siblings and required some basic discipline, but for the most part she was delightful and loving. She began kindergarten at Fort Worth County Day School, the excellent private preparatory school where her five brothers and sisters had graduated or were about to graduate. Toward the end of the first grade, her teacher, Mrs. Van Buskirk, who had also taught four of her siblings, informed me at a parent-teacher conference that Chelsea might be dyslexic. This was a surprise because Chelsea could read, although not very well, and because she was exceptionally bright. After appropriate professional testing, Mrs. Van Buskirk's years of experience proved correct. Chelsea was dyslexic as well as attention deficit. Chelsea and I were to learn much more about learning differences, but what it initially meant to us, after a psychologically hurtful second grade experience, was that Chelsea was not capable of keeping up with the rigorous demands of a traditional preparatory curriculum. It felt like failure to her to have to leave the school where her siblings could learn and compete.*

*She transferred to a specialized school for children with learning differences, Star Point. It was a wonderful place with exceptional teachers who made all the difference in Chelsea's wounded self-esteem and in her ability to read and learn, but at the time it felt to her like one more thing to be ashamed of. Initially we were given little hope that Chelsea would return to mainstream education, but before the school year was over, we were encouraged to let Chelsea try a loving as well as challenging school, All Saints Episcopal Day School. With many extra hours' work each day Chelsea not only kept up at All Saints, but she began to excel.*

*Looking back on Chelsea's extraordinary effort and the academic success she achieved despite her handicaps, I can see how they fit into her ability to pretend that everything was fine. In fact, she made us all believe that making good grades was her highest priority. In fact her highest priority was appearing to be the perfect child in order to hide her shame. Chelsea was running scared. Her fear was that we would remember or that someone would find out. The perfect pretender had her teachers, family, and friends all fooled. She even fooled herself. She had become an artist at running a subconscious scam. By overachieving, acting happy, and being popular she convinced us that she was the "best little girl in the world." Yet she always felt she was shamed. The grades, the awards, the invitations, the smiles were her ways of coping. They served as distractions from the growing, secret fear she held inside.*

*During these happy, successful years I did what I think most parents would do. I enjoyed! What a treat to go to her school and hear the compliments, the congratulations, the accolades. I never questioned whether this was too good to be true. My hands were full with other terrific children, a husband, and a career that, although part time, was really taking off. My position at the Parenting Guidance Center had led to the opportunity to appear weekly on the Metroplex NBC television news as their parenting adviser with parenting tips. This exposure led to regular guest appearances on the nationally syndicated television show "COPE," during which viewers called in with their family or parenting problems. After ten years on NBC and seven years on "COPE," I signed a contract with Taylor Publishing Company to write my first book,* The Overloving Parent, *which was published in 1992.*

*The point of this digression is to highlight the irony. I was supposed to be a parenting expert after all. I was introduced as such on television and at the numerous speeches I gave. I was always giving advice on how parents could improve their parenting skills and knowledge. I had six loving and responsible children and stepchildren, including Chelsea, who were increasing that sense of pride that I was a great mother with knowledge and experience to offer others. My children worked hard at making me look good. As they each moved through college and into adulthood, Bill and I took pride in their accomplishments, hard work, and success.*

*We were down to one child, Chelsea, living at home and in high school. This seemed so easy when we remembered the hectic days of parenting several teenagers at one time, with all their friends, sports, scholastic challenges, and extracurricular activities. How simple it was to have only one to emotionally support and encourage. Chelsea also made it a fun experience. From her first days in high school she continued to excel. She was on the honor roll taking honors classes, was a cheerleader, a member of student council, voted class favorite, played varsity basketball, and was involved in many clubs and school activities. Again we enjoyed it all. Bill and I had always gone to all the children's performances and competitions. Now we had only one beautiful adolescent to watch and it was more rewarding than ever. We knew how fast the opportunities to be with a child ended.*

*Then near the end of Chelsea's sophomore year, when she seemed to be the happiest, most successful teenager imaginable, she made the strangest request. Chelsea asked to go to boarding school for her last two years of high school. Remember, Chelsea struggled with learning differences and attention deficit, putting in many extra hours to maintain her A average. A boarding school would be even more challenging. She would also be giving up a secure place of achievement and social success as well as strong bonds of friendship she had with many lifelong friends. We also had a wonderful and close relationship. Being so much younger than her siblings, Chelsea had been like an only child in many ways for the past seven years. She had tons of attention from Bill and me, as well as from her grandparents, who saw her several times a week as well as attended many of her events.*

*Chelsea's argument, which she felt strongly about and we eventually accepted, was that she wanted a better education and that only at a competitive preparatory boarding school could she be truly prepared for a great college experience. I hoped it would be a phase, that after visiting schools in the Northeast, she would be satisfied with staying in high school in Fort Worth. To the contrary, Chelsea was impressed with the schools she chose to visit and she seemed more determined than ever to spend her junior and senior years in a prestigious boarding school in Connecticut.*

*After tearful good-byes her junior year in high school to dear friends and family, Chelsea and I left for a few days in New York City and then on to Connecticut where we set her up in the dorm room that was to be her home away from home for the next two years. Chelsea seemed to be more fragile than I had ever seen her. We had always been close, but she had never had a problem going off to camp or taking trips away from me. This boarding school experience was her idea and choice, yet as it came time for me to spend the night in a quaint bed and breakfast before I headed back to Texas, she insisted on spending the night with me. The next morning she seemed faint and extremely weak. She said she did not know if she could stay at the school. I encouraged her to give it a try for one semester, then she could always come home. I thought it was normal fear of a new environment and truly expected her to be one of the most popular young women on campus within the week. She had always adapted well and met challenges with incredible determination.*

*Later that morning, as I said good-bye to her at her dorm, she could not stop crying. I thought her tears were like mine, filled with a combination of love and grief. I was going to miss Chelsea so much. Most parents prepare to release a child to college and adult life, but this was two years too early. As much as I wanted for Chelsea what she seemed to want for herself—the best education possible—it felt like too great a sacrifice. I was forfeiting two precious years with her for an education that would prepare her for success in college. It was a sad, difficult day. Somehow I took photographs of her in front of her dorm, kept saying encouraging words, and promised she could come home after just one semester, hoping she would still want to come home.*

*Before I boarded my flight home, I called Chelsea from La Guardia Airport. Instead of hearing her positive, upbeat voice, she could not stop crying. She pleaded with me to return and take her home. One of the hardest things I have ever done was to tell her to give it a try for a semester and then come home. On the flight home I replayed our trip to the school, our conversations, her weak physical condition that morning. Most of all I heard a desperation in her cries for me to bring her home. I prayed for Chelsea and I prayed for the wisdom to know the right thing to do.*

*That evening, emotionally drained, I joined Bill in our bedroom and described in detail the last forty-eight hours. This was a Chelsea I had never experienced. She had always been so brave, so enthusiastic about facing the many challenges throughout her sixteen years. Reluctantly and anxiously I called her again. Chelsea was hysterical about how she had to come home. She had to convince me. She was desperate, so she began to pour out the truth.*

*I don't remember her exact words, but what she confessed was that she was bulimic. She probably did not give me many details, such as the fact that she had been bulimic for almost a year. What I remember most was fear for Chelsea along with the simultaneous but conflicting feelings of shock and, "Aha! This makes sense." On the one hand I was wondering how I could have missed the signs of an eating disorder. On the other hand I began to see how all the things I had wondered and worried about fell into place. First of all her decision to go away to school was not just about having a better education. Chelsea explained that she hoped leaving the socially competitive high school environment she had been in would help her overcome her bulimia. To the contrary, being away from home in a new environment without friends and family caused her bulimia to accelerate out of control. As her departure for boarding school had neared, her purging episodes had increased. In the twenty-four hours she had been on the boarding school campus, she realized the mistake of trying to run from her problem. The moving solution had backfired.*

*I must say something about Chelsea's body weight here, because that is what everyone assumes should be the red flag that a person has an eating disorder. All through middle school Chelsea had been an ideal size and weight. She was very shapely at an early age. The summer before high school she had put on a few unwanted pounds, nothing to be concerned about but not the weight at which she wanted to enter high school. To adults she looked terrific, but to Chelsea and probably many of her peers she needed to drop about five pounds. She went to aerobics regularly and tried to cut back her calories, but the pounds did not fall off. I thought she looked beau-*

*tiful and never suggested that she should lose weight. But I knew she was unhappy.*

*Sometime between her freshman and sophomore year, she began to lose weight. She was exercising a little more and watching her fat intake more. I never knew the exact number of pounds she lost and would not have considered asking because I did not want to focus on weight. There was certainly nothing to be alarmed about; there was not a dramatic weight loss. My best guess would be that she lost between five and ten pounds. She went from a size eight to a size six, which was a little thin for her 5 foot 8 inch height, but compared to her classmates she was not too thin. Most of the girls had less mature figures, lacking Chelsea's curves. Chelsea looked beautiful and healthy. Friends frequently commented on her great looks as well as her other much more important inner qualities.*

*What I now understand is that an eating disorder is not about weight, nor is weight a sure indicator that there is a problem. Chelsea looked great, but she was spiraling toward death in an out-of-control disease.*

*By the time we got to New York the few days before we went to the boarding school, Chelsea had become very picky about where she would eat, finding very few restaurants that offered "healthy" menu items. I remember walking around Soho with her, both of us tired and hungry, unable to find a place to have lunch that offered something she would eat. On the one hand I admired her will power and "healthy" attitude, while on the other hand I worried that she would not be able to find the low-fat food she insisted on at the boarding school. Now her excessive concern with food was making sense. Chelsea had an eating disorder. As I learned more about eating disorders over the next few years, I realized there had been many warning signs that I had missed. The guilt was just beginning to strangle me.*

*The decision for Chelsea to leave the boarding school was not reached lightly but reasonably quickly and with professional advice. The night I returned from Connecticut and heard Chelsea's tearful confession, I called her father in L.A. He and his wife discussed with me all the ramifications of Chelsea giving up the opportunity of attending a great school as well as her physical and psychological conditions. Chelsea began classes, the school was alerted to her bulimia and her desire to leave, and we all continued to talk by phone frequently the first few days of school. Finally the level of Chelsea's desperation was realized when she tried to run away from school, the most uncharacteristic act I could imagine at that time. Chelsea's dad and stepmother flew to Connecticut and took her to a highly respected psychiatrist in Manhattan. The psychiatrist's recommendation was that Chelsea had a better chance of recovering from bulimia in the safety and familiarity of her home. After less than a week at boarding school, Chelsea was returning home. I was so relieved. I was positive that in my arms she could heal. How prideful of me to think I could make her well. How ignorant of me to think I could help her control a disease that was all about the need to feel self-control.*

# Part Three: 18 Years Old

❦❦

*To live is to suffer, to survive is to find meaning in the suffering. If there is a purpose in life at all, there must be a purpose in suffering.*
—ALLPORT

# Summer 1994

*Letter to a Friend,*

I write you now not in condemnation but in truth. I doubt I will ever understand your vindictive motives. I loved you more than life itself. That you were my best friend is far too trite a statement and could never reveal my passion for our life-binding relationship.

I don't believe in coincidence. You found me coiled in pain, a confusion of tears, ones that fought to come. The touch of your hand I never saw, but I was calmed by your presence. I knew you were there and my pain seemed to disappear.

I prayed every night that God would not be so cruel as to take away the only person I truly loved. I knew without you I would be empty. All the holes you filled would be cold and dark. I would steep in pain. I never wanted to see what was really there. You protected me. You met me in triumph with praise like no other. You stole my dreams of a painful death for a moment. You tried so hard to help me forget what had always been. I thought I could never have enough of you. An intimate relationship was much too simple. I wanted us to be one. I became you and you me. How could you be my hope and my desire for life? I gave you my heart and my mind. But never could you have my spirit. Every night I wanted so to give that to you, but you never would surrender.

I hated that little voice, weakly crying, and it only got louder and louder. We fought so hard. We fought with my life to kill that crying spirit that we could not claim. You lied to me. You promised so much. You promised the world. I didn't care, even when I knew I still tried to make our union perfect.

Our relationship will ultimately perish. I could say that I have never truly felt hate. Saying you hate another is different than living hate. I live with the most insidious hate every day of my life. I do not claim to be a victim who has fallen prey to this disease. I was the fool who made the choice. Words could never do you justice. The amazing but terrifying reality is that my deep-rooted hatred pales in comparison to your ability to rip another's soul, mind, and spirit. This pain will linger, hitting deep in a place I never knew existed. The hard truth is that this war is within me. But this hatred could be my salvation. You are not my destiny. The mystery of my life sustains me now. I won't ask why me, but I will come to understand what is, and what has made you part of me.

∽⌒⌒∾

I am awakened by the voice I loathe. You call me early in the morning. You tell me this is your day. "Look in the mirror," you say. "It won't take long to see the faults. If you believe they are merely faults, you are just lying. Look again. Now do you see? It's the truth. It's the way you are. Did you really think I would let you rise without your glasses? Turn to the big mirror. Pinch it, make it worse, but really there is no need. You can see your fat, and you can see it grow.

"Yes, that's right, begin to recall all the sins that touched your lips. Now you can see that you shall pay for your weakness. Don't make excuses. A day without physical purging (exercise)? Who are you fooling? It is black and white. You're not good enough. Hey, where do you think you are going? Look at all the bumps and imperfections on your skin. Get rid of them. Who cares if it hurts? You deserve it. You have been bad. Search, look harder, fix it. You can move on when you see the blood.

"Run your fingers down your thighs. Turn to the side. Don't you see they are growing? If you look like this now you are going to look more like shit with each year. Who would want you then? You won't even be able to stand yourself. A worthless woman without a decent body. No one will care. The only attention you will receive is the remembrance of the way you were. 'Look how she let herself go. Remember when she gained all that weight when she needed to lose weight? In fact, she was fat. Poor Chelsea, she couldn't control her weight. She is not important. You know that's so true.' When you begin to lose your body you have no worth, no purpose, no credibility. You are bad and disgusting. You will never be on top. You know it's true. Pick at yourself some more. It might hurt, but you're gross, you have got to get it out. You have to be better. Look what you have done to your legs. Yeah, but who cares? Your pain is worth it. It is fun to hurt yourself. Come on, admit it. You are lost without me. You hate yourself so much, but I am always here and always will be. I only want the best for you. I want you to be perfect. You and I are all you need. Let's stay alone tonight. We can cook together after aerobics. You can come home to the place that is the safest for you. You can hide us from your friends, but you and I will know how good it will feel and how relieved you will be. All alone, just you and me. That's right. Give in. It's long overdue. What is one time, just one fix?"

∞∞

My response to the talk I hear:

I hate you so fucking much. You have been really strong for a while. Not today. This is bullshit. You are lies, all lies.

Listen and hear me because I tell you the truth. I love myself. I am beautiful inside and out. Furthermore, I am God's child and have no need for you. I do not need to torture my body this way. I believe in Jesus and believe in his plan for my life. My heart is alive; my hope is strong. Through my tribulation I grow closer to the Lord and I become stronger and more alive. I love making people laugh and smile. I love people and being with people. Now I can repay the joy. I, Chelsea Browning Smith, want to live the adventure, always knowing I will never be given more than I can bear. I love to talk with people, my friends, and just hang out. God gave me this body and these trials for a reason. I know his way will be done in my life. Yes, I am kicking ass. You can go straight back to hell where you started. I want you to die, you evil, lying, deceitful, disgusting, little bitch.

∞∞

I hate the weight I am. I look huge. I am really fighting my symptoms. I would love to restrict and lose weight. I can't stand this. I have been coming up with ways of not eating. I see things black or white. Yesterday Bret and I talked about staying together and how I need to just go to school and not worry about things here. I don't want to eat. I told myself all day I was getting too big! I felt uncomfortable all day. It is amazing all the ways I try to weenie out of my obligation to my recovery, and I try to control situations and my feelings. I am so quick to focus on food or obsess about my body rather than focus on reality. I place so many unrealistic expectations on others. I look to my relationships to fulfill my self-centered needs and expectations. That's not fair to the person because only I can effectively meet my needs. I can't fix others, and they can't fix me. I can't change time, and most of all I can't lie to myself, believing in my will and desire to control my weight.

∞∞

Mom really got to me yesterday. The main way she expresses her love is through catering to our every need. It gets old. She is such a suck-up. I hate it. I get angry when she is trying so hard to be nice and helpful. I find it is easy to walk all over her when she does that. I just hate the fact that she walks around on eggshells. It's like she is thinking, "Let's not upset the identified patient," as though I am going to crack at any moment. She wants to make everything so perfect for me, which is wonderful but not realistic. I want her to be real and get mad or tired like any mom. Also, I hate how she watches me and tries to pretend that she doesn't.

∞∞

Lauren and I have the cutest room. I wanted John Holt to take me to Austin and move me in. I asked Mom not to come. I hope she is relieved. Today is the first day of classes. I feel calm and clear this morning. It scares me that I don't want to let go of my desire to be in Fort Worth. This move is really scary. I just left a treatment center three month ago, and here I am living in a new city, with new people (except for Lauren and Elizabeth). But the changes are hard. The first thing I need to do is find a support group and a therapist. I am so scared of losing what feels right and good. Is that so crazy?

∞∞

I want to live for today. I find myself thinking more about going home to visit. I am trying to cheat on my eating. I don't want to gain weight. That is a lie. I don't want to do this, the lies, the preoccupation and avoidance of my fear. This is all so overwhelming. I don't want to get out of touch. I guess I am really restricting. There are girls with eating disorders in this dorm. It is amazing how prevalent eating disorders are. It is also sad that they are ignored—even accepted. I like living with Lauren. Having her know my stuff and being able to talk to her is so helpful. She really tries to understand. The classes are really hard and huge. Math is impossible. You have to be a brain to understand at such a rapid pace.

∞∞

God, I am in pain. What is going on? I want to say I can't do this, but I think I am choosing not to do this. I don't want this. I wanted to wait and come in August like every other college student. I was not ready for another major change this soon. I was the one who wanted to come here. No one made me. I can't see the good that lies beyond my fear of what I think might happen.

I am simply existing. The bad stuff is coming out. I feel like shit. I can't give up. I am such a quitter. I am gaining weight, my clothes are tighter, and I look awful. I would have left a long time ago if I thought people wouldn't care, but what would they all think? That's just it. I don't know what the hell I want or what I am doing or anything else. I feel like I am just waiting for time to pass. That to me is death. There is no worse way to live. To just wait and want time to pass. Why do I think so much, constantly feeling and changing? I am one big adjustment. I don't know where, what, or how I am suppose to do this. God, I want to tell you that I don't think you care and that you are not a very good listener. I wish I could make you show me where to go next. I am so clueless. I am pleading with you to help me. I am drowning, I can't feel like this. It kills me when I think you are distant. Please, my heart is becoming callused and I am shutting down. Why am I choosing not to feel your presence Lord? Word for today: release.

∞∞

I am sitting here by myself. I just finished eating at Taco Cabana. I want to throw up. I just feel so full. I look at myself in the mirror, and my neck and face are growing. I am scared. I am really scared. It would be so easy to just let it out—so easy. No one would know. God give me the strength. Please give me the courage to trust what I don't know. I do not have to throw up. Throwing up is not something a normal person would do. My mind is telling me something is wrong. I don't buy that, but I need to wait. I need to be patient and just wait, just wait it out. I hate the support group meetings here. In all honesty I have not really given them a chance. I have been so anxious today. This is such bullshit. I am running scared. This won't fix any of my problems. Why does it appear to be the perfect solution? Maybe I could just eat less tomorrow. I am struggling to see things clearly. I am so preoccupied. Here it goes again, this racing in my mind, desperately trying to make a plan for tomorrow. Sorting the chaos in my mind, trying to make sense of anything and everything. I am drowning in this madness. "I will not eat this." "I better do this." "What if this happens tomorrow?" "Oh, I walked today, that makes it better." "I don't have to be so hard on myself. I got some of the calories out."

Maybe I need to realize no matter where I live or what I do my recovery and healing process must take precedence over everything. No matter what, it will not be easy. I had no idea recovery would be as crazy as, if not crazier than, the eating disorder itself. I am choosing to immerse myself in lies. Why could I not choose to live the truth, to just try to live the truth? The other way is not working. Okay, what do I know to be true in my life? I have curly brown hair, I am five-foot-eight, with green eyes, olive skin, straight teeth, and I am in recovery. I am grateful I can separate the lies from the truth. I just resisted throwing up when it felt like the only way. Now there is the truth.

I miss feeling love. I don't cry much, even though I feel all the things that could make a person cry. I am going to tell Lauren how I freaked out the other day. I started trying on her clothes to see if she is that much skinnier that I am. I told myself that if I could wear her clothes, I would be okay. That is crazy. Even when I was at my lowest weight she had the smallest waist, and there was no way in hell her clothes would ever fit. I need to make amends to her. I am so embarrassed to admit it to her. That's real smooth Chelsea. I am really sorry Lauren. I love you so much and you have been my best friend since birth. I don't want to bring you into this. I would never want to hurt you. I did not mean to be disloyal. I didn't mean for my screwed-up neurotic obsession to get in the way, but I guess that happened a long time ago. It doesn't excuse my act, but that voice wouldn't shut up.

Lauren is the best. She has stuck by me through all this stuff. I can't imagine how hard and frustrating it must be for someone who has not been here to understand or know how to help. I am grateful for her sake that she does not wake to the redundant, constant nagging voice that I wake up to almost every day of my life. Lauren does the best thing for me. She listens well and often. Lauren's concern is always explained through love. She loves me in her own way, and she is consistent. I will never be able to repay her. Lauren is a true friend and I am blessed.

There is this tutoring center where most of the students in the provisional program go for help. A tutor named Lee works there. I feel so uncomfortable around him. He is from someplace in Britain and is about twenty-eight. He gives me the creeps. I will look up from my work and he will be staring at me. He favors me in the class and always wants to talk to me before, after, and during. Lee is not nerdy. He just has this staring problem. He seems manipulative. He corners me and takes up a ton of time. He is also dominating, sort of slimy, and I don't trust him.

∞∞

This week is going to be one of the hardest, and I don't want to do it. I have two tests and a paper due. I need to make allowance for the fact that I am not perfect, remembering all the while I am human, not the best and not the worst. Remuda wasn't lying when they said, "If you thought your eating disorder was hard, try recovery." They could not have stressed enough how hard recovery really is. I am amazed sometimes at my ability to hang on when there is nothing but the will that says to hang on. When I focus on food and how much I hate my body, life quickly becomes just that small and insignificant, and my world that lifeless. Sometimes in the heart of my eating disorder I would try to remember what I felt like and how I thought before I got sick. But I couldn't remember, so then I would think of someone I admired not for their physical appearance but for their mind, hope, peace, and love of life. When I looked at the big picture, I knew that I wanted a healthy and loving life. I never lost the hope that my life was created for more than where I was taking it. I want more, and any person can see that anyone deserves more than the life I was choosing to giving myself. Holding on to an idea and a goal bigger than me will keep me safe in recovery.

I think I inherited dreaming—the belief that I can do anything—from my Dad. I know no one is going to do this for me. No one else can bail me out or live recovery for me. It's all me; it's all about me. I cannot continue to focus on the small symptoms of the disease that are right in front of me. I pray that the worrying about whether and when the symptoms will leave will cease. They are painful, but in the midst of it all I miss the life. I am missing my life, the one I am strong enough to live. I don't know when I began this war with myself, but it has caused me to fear myself. It's caused me to doubt any deeper level of self-understanding and my ability to take care of myself. I cringe at the thought of what lies below the unturned surface, that which grips my mind and transcends all awareness of reality. It's waiting to take me under.

I pray, Lord, that I am silent long enough to hear your voice, long enough to inhabit your will. I don't think I need to understand you because I know that you understand me. Thank you for this peace and helping me through the struggles. Word for the day: understanding.

∞∞

Living with so many girls, it is easy to get sucked into all sorts of stuff—the conversations about the "need" for fat-free everything, the constant condemning of the meal that they ate the night before, the complaints that they already have so much cellulite. These conversations have always taken place inside my head. but to hear them going on around me and hear all these girls obsessing about their bodies and food drives me crazy. I can't help but think I need to think like that. That is their norm and I cannot let that be mine. For now I am not ready to be around people who are into that stuff. I don't want to be around it any more than I have to. My life is so different in some ways from most college girls. Our thoughts might be too similar to discern an obvious difference, but my loaded thoughts are now labeled. I know that my choices must be different than in the past. I don't resent the fact that my choices are different. In some ways I feel lucky because they too are running a race I once believed I had to win in order to live. I was grasping for the quick fix, trying to find happiness in places where happiness was never meant to be. I know society is going more and more in the opposing direction. Rarely do I turn on the TV or radio without hearing weight as a topic for a commercial, talk show, or sitcom. Being bitter toward it all is not rational, nor is the expectation that women will not worry and talk about their weight. I need to protect myself and understand the role I choose for weight and exercise to play in my life. The obsession is not my duty anymore. I know my fixation was never meant to and never will fix my internal needs. My fall was inevitable.

∞·∞

It's unbelievable all that has gone on this weekend. I am blown away. Yesterday I was in so much pain, I truly did not want to live anymore. I was so miserable. I felt as though my world was falling apart. Let me back up. I am not going to be at UT after this summer. The math class that was a required part of the provisional program was way too hard. I was failing it, and the professor told me I was not going to pass. The class would be a failing grade on my transcript. Well, I might have jumped the gun when I took it upon myself to drop the class, which meant I could not go to school here in the fall. My mom flipped out. Yelling, she told me, "Don't think you are coming home. You are staying in Austin and finishing the rest of the courses you are signed up for." I about died. For the first time in my life she was not on my side, and furthermore, she was pissed. If I had made Mom mad, Dad would disown me. I am choosing to wait to tell him. My quick decision means I might not be with my two best friends, Lauren and Elizabeth. They are doing better than I am and might pass all the classes. No matter how hard I scream and cry, nothing is going to change my choice. I think I screwed up. I know I would not have passed though. I failed all three tests and got ninety percent wrong on every homework assignment. I can't stand having Mom abandon me like this. I have never made her this mad.

∞

My body is moving so fast with all I am trying to do and my mind is doing its best to beat it. Last night I went for ice cream. It was great. Then it hit, and my mind has not stopped since. I am scared. I am terrified. I feel so pressured to go exercise and get the calories nullified. I am doing, doing, doing, and want all this material stuff in the hope that it will make me feel better. It is so hard sometimes to just walk away from my desires and wants.

If I understand my eating disorder as the disease it is and look at my cravings and urges as painful symptoms, it makes a little more sense. Think about this: If I am dying to eat a whole piece of cake, I hold back, telling myself instead, "Later when you are alone." Or I tell myself not to eat all my dinner, thinking, "Later I can get something that I really want to fill me up." Compare this to having a sore throat. What do I do to fix that? Well, I take Advil, throat spray, and gargle with saltwater. I don't give those steps a second thought. I do what it takes to stop the pain. When the pain starts I don't try to figure out how I could have caught a sore throat, I just take action. So when my eating disorder symptoms occur, why not handle them just like any other physical discomfort? I have specific ways to alleviate the pain and ultimately change the course of the symptoms' path. I eat my meal, period. I just do it. There is none of this "later on I can eat what I really want" talk, fantasizing about what I could do with food or what I could just have a bit of, or a taste of. I just eat my meal and go on, not dragging it out.

Chelsea, most of all you have to be realistic. You are an

eating-disordered person in recovery. You're not playing with the same cards as everyone else. I will not make myself crazy by repeatedly trying solutions that have proven themselves unsuccessful. If something isn't working I will step back and wait for guidance.

∞∞

I talked with Molly last night. It makes me sad because she sounds just like I did. Daily I get calls from another girl who has started talking about her problem or a parent who is finally accepting that there is something wrong with a daughter. Eating disorders are more prevalent than I want to believe. It's like an epidemic; it's become the trendy thing to do. I wish I could catch them all before they fall into their emptiness and obsessive insanity. I wish they knew what I now do. They are all playing a game they will never win.

After seeing girls succeed and not succeed I've thought a lot about what it takes to be successful in recovery. Women who have been addicts for a long time naturally will have a harder time choosing recovery and staying in recovery. I believe that within every eating-disordered person there is an imaginary line that she cannot see. She is unaware of its beginning or end. For some women, finding this limit happens fast. They play with eating disorder behavior for a while and for whatever reason are able to walk away and put the fixation behind them. Others hit it hard. Ignoring their hearts and denying their hopes, they become even more attached to the obsessive symptoms. They continue in their rituals, because now they believe the rituals are a means of survival, a lifestyle. When they look in the mirror, they only see parts. No longer are their bodies whole. By some rare chance if they catch reality and see the whole picture, they don't even recognize it. The addiction is so intense that what was once a distraction or a healthy choice to lose weight now causes their souls to ebb. They get wrapped up in themselves. Their identities become the disease. They cross the line, and for most, to some degree it's for life.

I am not saying some won't get better or go in and out of recovery, but someone achieving full recovery, a sheer freedom, is not common; in fact, I think it is rare. To me the saddest part is the choice they had but never chose to see. They never saw that there really was another way to cope with life. I am not saying that I am healed, nor am I saying my recovery has been perfect. Rather, I know all these things to be true because I've lived them. Everyone is different in their pursuit of and needs in recovery. I do believe in finding a common ground and discovering some basic truth in this disease, even if it is learning from another woman what not to do. Each story has its own twist, its own unique qualities, but when you get to the heart of each girl, the stories are chillingly similar. I wish I had the answer for them, but I don't have it for me yet.

One thing I do know and believe with all my heart, is that no woman is forced to live her life with an eating disorder. She may die trying to find a way out, but if she wants it badly enough, if she wants to live no matter the cost, and if she is determined not to die, she can live and she will. I believe there is much more to say about this disease than being a mere victim of its suffocating, baffling obsession. Now, I can see how a woman with a feeding tube down her throat would have a hard time agreeing (or thinking for that matter), but at some point she can choose to believe that she deserves more in life and that in fact, she deserves to live. I don't think I am lucky. God has blessed me, but I have been open to him. I am grateful for my place and success in recovery. I don't know what has helped make it click for me. Even though I struggle a lot, going back and forth, I never forget that I deserve more. I want more, and I believe there is more.

God, however you want to use me please show me, because I am open. Rick (my therapist in Austin) told me something really cool: I don't have trouble finding myself; I struggle with accepting what I find.

∞∞

I leave for Phoenix today. I am so excited. Lee from the tutoring center totally freaked me out before I left. While walking me out to my car he asked all these questions about where I was going, why, and with whom. When I told him I was going to see my boyfriend, I thought that would make him leave me alone, but it made him want more. He opened my door and stood there telling me not to make any mistakes I would regret. He told me how I could not trust Bret and that there would always be something waiting here for me when I got back. I was like, "Okay, have a good Fourth of July." He wouldn't shut up. He was so redundant. Finally he let me go. Then while Lauren and I were packing, getting ready to leave, the phone rang. It was Lee. I wanted to know how in the hell he got my number, because all of ours are unlisted. He started telling me again to be careful and that I shouldn't do anything I would regret. Then he sort of apologized for getting too much into my business and then finished the conversation by wishing me a great Fourth. He added that when I got back, he and I would have to go get a drink together. All the girls started freaking out that he had called. We figured he must have looked in the files at the tutoring center to get my number. I thought it was creepy.

After I returned from a great weekend with Bret, Lee offered to arrange an outside tutoring session to tutor my class, which consists of six guys and me, at one of the guys' houses at midnight. I thought, fine. But after class he stopped me, once again wanting to arrange a separate private session. He has been telling me for a while that he would help me outside of school

138

but not to let the tutoring center know. I thought that was a little strange, but fine. He suggested some places, but I didn't feel comfortable with them. In the end, I felt safest asking him to just come to my dorm around 2:00 P.M. I said we could work for an hour studying for my biology test. He came, and we studied in the breakfast room. It seemed perfectly innocent, and he told me I could just pay him later. I told him that I had to make a B in the class and that I was really scared because I didn't know the information well enough. In his little British accent told me that if I do what he says and work really hard I can make an A because I am so smart. He then offered to help me at the tutoring place later that night said that the only opening he had was around 11:00 P.M. I thought this was perfect—a well populated, neutral place. So I went.

When I got there he met me in the lobby and we went upstairs to this small tutoring room. I started opening my books, immediately trying to focus on the material and questions. We had not been there ten minutes when another tutor came into the room asking Lee to turn off all the lights after he locked up. I thought, "Holy shit, here we are all alone and this Lee can do whatever he wants. I was so nervous. He then tells me not to be scared and that he can tell I am holding things back from him. He really just wants to get to know me better, he said, because I am so intelligent and kind. This did not help my fear, and he could tell I was scared. It didn't help that I could not answer one of the questions he asked. I told him I was just burnt out and that I wanted to go. Lee told me to wait because he wanted to walk me to my car. Knowing the path back was dark and much longer than I wanted to be alone with him, I assured him I was fine. Of course, he insisted I wait. He opened my car door and talked for a while. I have no clue what he said, but he wants to get to know me better, to go have a drink—he loves whisky.

He asked whether I was going to the off-campus study section tomorrow night. "Yes," I said, and I shut the door. He gives me the creeps but I want to do well on the test and to prove that I can handle this whole thing.

∽

I don't even want to retell last night. It doesn't matter. I won't forget it for a long time. I went for about twenty minutes to the study session, and they were not studying so I left. As I was leaving I handed Lee the ten dollars everyone had agreed on. He gave me this look like I was completely insulting him. He grabbed my hand and said, "Don't you dare pay me." I acted calm and said, "Okay, well I'm going back to study." Later, Lauren and I were talking in our room, and our friends were coming in and out. I told them the latest update with Lee, and they were freaked. It was about 2:00 a.m. when the phone rang. It was Lee. He sounded weird and said he was downstairs and wanted to talk to me. So all the girls freaked and followed me downstairs. There the weirdo was in the lobby, and he asked me to go outside with him. They told me not to, but the badass that I wanted to be decided to go anyway. He said in this furious tone, "I know you have something to tell me." Right then I knew what he had heard—that I was not going to school here next year. He was so pissed. He wanted to know why and kept pressuring me to stop withholding information from him, that he could tell that I was in a lot of pain. He kept trying to get me to disclose things to him. Then he told me I was special, so different from the other girls, and how smart I was.

Then he said for the second time, "Let's take a walk." I said, "No, I like it here." He promised me he would not hurt me. He just wanted to get away from all this "bullshit I had been living in." Finally I told him that he did not know the whole story and that I was taking care of myself by not staying.

I simply said I was in recovery from anorexia and bulimia. I was under too much pressure. The first thing out of his mouth was, "Who hurt you so much that you would torture yourself like that? Please, let's get away from here so we can talk." His voice got more demanding, and he kept on repeating, "You are so wounded. Who has hurt you? What happened to you when you were a child?" I swear it was like he knew that I had been sexually abused, and I guess he thought that if he could get me to open up that he would have me then. I stood my ground.

Then the game changed. He asked me to sit on the steps because he wanted to tell me something that he had never told anyone other than his parents. He asked me if I could see the bald spot on his head. I replied, yes, and then he said that when he was sixteen he was put into a mental institution for three years and doesn't remember anything. All the drugs he was on caused his hair to fall out. At some point in the conversation I zoned out. I felt like I was suffocating and that I had to get out of there. All I could think was how badly I did not want to know this crap about my tutor. This was my freaking biology tutor. What the hell was going on.

In the midst of his vomiting of horrific details from the insane asylum I said, "Lee, I have got to go," and ran for the door. All of my friends were standing there with their noses pressed to the window. They had been waiting the whole hour we were outside. I just kept running. I thought I was going to suffocate. I was shaking all over and completely freaked. Lauren grabbed me and put her arms around me. I just burst into tears. It was awful. I hate him so much. He tried so hard to get into my mind and I thought the whole time I was in control. I had no idea that his motives were so evil, and I know that if I had I taken that walk he would have raped me. I felt like my mind had been raped and filled with all this sick stuff. I had no control, except when I got the hell away from him.

Model mugging taught me how to defend myself physically, but the physical also trained me mentally. I believed I had a right to say I had had enough and that I owed him nothing, not even my time. I am so grateful for the confidence that one weekend gave me. Lee was so much smarter than the psycho stereotype. I feel fortunate. The whole situation could have left a greater mark on my life. I hate him so much. I might sound dramatic, but for some reason I am so scared now that he will find me alone and I will not have a way out. I am going to stay the hell away from him. All the girls were so sweet and even the guys had noticed that he was really stepping over the line with me. It just makes me so sick to think about the way he would reach for my hand or touch me. He was really smart and knew what he was doing. I told Mom, and everyone thinks I should report him.

∞∞

This new way of looking at others' perceptions of me is unbelievable. I love it. I learned that the way others look at me, what they think of me, and how they see me is a reflection of them, not me. I can't believe I have wasted so much of my life trying to predict and control what others think of me, how they see me, or how they feel about me. God, I am going nuts. Please help me feel what loving myself is like. I don't know how to be okay and to accept what is. I want so much to accept who you have made. When I get into fear and feel a strong need to be accepted and to prove myself, I will first see if I have accepted that which I fear within myself.

∞∞

My Lord if my life is going to be constantly thinking, feeling, and up and down all the time, then I don't want to live. I don't like feeling so much. I can get so upset and into myself. I

DIARY OF AN EATING DISORDER

desperately try to figure out what is wrong, what the answer is, and why I can't fix my pain. I want to scream. I am exhausted. Please, I am begging you to please release me from these burdens, I am carrying around so much weight on my shoulders. I can hardly bear it anymore. I feel up and down all the time. I constantly question my choices, moods, emotions, weight, and purpose. I feel as though I am a little kid without a parent leading me. I try to understand how to live in a way that is so foreign to me. I guess when everyone else was learning that stuff I was in aerobics class. They tell me these feelings are all normal, but it doesn't mean they are pleasant. I can't experience the good without also living the bad. I am so grateful for my friends. They really help me see things that I could never see in myself, like my being successful and that I am a hard worker. Next time I write I hope things will be better.

∞∞

Brad told one of his friends that I was in recovery from an eating disorder. That is fine, but his friend Matt caught me totally off guard asking me about it. I am on this trip with all these people, including Matt (Brad's friend), and he won't quit watching me eat. It's like he is waiting for me to scarf up everything on the table and his plate too, then throw up right in front of everyone. I might throw up on him if he doesn't leave me alone. I am not some freak in the circus.

∞∞

Rick (my counselor) and I have been working on my relationship with my sister, Ashley. He gave me an assignment to call her and ask what it was like growing up in our house and then to just listen. Rick has also asked me to pray for her. Rick explained to me that by looking at life through her eyes and experiences, I might understand her more and better understand where she is coming from. So much of the anger I feel toward my sister comes from things I struggle with in myself. In many ways she represents what I won't accept as part of me. Seeing her represent parts of myself scare me.

I am wearing this rubber band and around my wrist. I am to pop myself every time I think about food, tell myself bad stuff about my body, or have obsessive thoughts. It is starting to hurt and my wrist is getting red.

∞∞

Today is a good day! Last night I talked to Matt (relapse therapist) from Remuda. He told me that I was the only patient he knew of that had not thrown up over the first six months after discharge. I was so happy. I have one week left here in Austin. I want to hug the world right now I am so happy.

∞∞

I have this crazy notion that if I eat what I want to, I will have the same body as my sister. I think exercising gets my mind started in that losing-weight cycle. I had to fix my body from the alcohol I drank last night. Save me. Give me a different way to see things. I know I am capable.

I can't believe I am going home tomorrow. We gave it a good try. Believe me I never thought that all three of us would end up at TCU together. I am so happy I am going to be with Lauren and Elizabeth.

∞∞

It doesn't get much better than this. It is Saturday morning. I am sitting alone in my house staring out a window. The sun is so beautiful. My huge cappuccino and classical music make my life complete. God gives me these moments to maintain my sanity. Lately I have been so grateful that I have God.

Without him I know I wouldn't want to continue pursuing recovery. Nor would I begin to know how to.

When I went shopping the other day, I was so frustrated because the clothes I want to fit don't, and I want them to so badly. I am struggling to accept my body and to believe I am not the size on the label but a person with feelings and a healthy body. But I don't have clothes to wear that fit.

I am so excited about starting TCU. I really can't wait.

∞∞

I don't know why I am up so early but I knew I didn't want to stay asleep. I am ready to get going. I hate the size I am. It drives me crazy. Maybe I am really scared and nervous about the first day of college and my weight is much easier to focus on than all the unknowns of school and the self-assigned expectations of my performance there.

Feelings are not always fact. My emotions are not factual, nor are they stable enough for me to act on.

What is so scary about loving and accepting myself? While moving into the dorm I found some old pictures. I started looking at these pictures of myself just seven months ago. I looked really scary and gross. I was so unattractive in these pictures. What did I do to myself? What will keep me from doing it again? I truly never saw myself the way I can see myself now in those pictures.

∞∞

Here I am again, same spot, different day, and different state. God, thank you. My feelings did change. I feel calm. I am glad today is Sunday and that I am going to church. I remember when I used to dread going. I didn't want to have any contact with God. I feared his ability to take my anorexia away, sentencing me to a life of fat forever. I just wanted him to leave me alone and not shake my little world of control.

∞∞

I am on my way to my favorite place, the lake. John, John Holt, Todd, and Jeff will be there. Since I was five, my family has spent every summer weekend at the lake. I grew up in awe of how cool my brothers and their friends were. In my eyes, their footsteps were golden. I ran with them everywhere, never thinking twice about my presence. I listened intently to every word and story about the girls they knew, vowing to do things differently, to be the type of girl they would love. I figured they must have known I was listening simply because they let me stay. Maybe they thought hearing their words and stories would help protect me from boys as I got older or to be a more attractive girl to boys.

Aside from John Holt I have never talked with them about my eating disorder. I have heard they can't comprehend why I would do that and how they don't understand eating disorders. I am ashamed to face them. I feel like I've let them down. During my disease they were some of the few people that made me want to let go of it. We have so much fun together. All we do is laugh and tease one another. Always they have loved me just like I am, and I know they couldn't care less what I look like. They just want me to be healthy and have me around to tease. I love them so much. I hope they know how much I have always idolized them, even though we are older now and do not talk about stuff like that. I will always know they would do anything for me. They made me believe I was wonderful in their eyes.

# *Fall 1994*

I hate fucking eating disorders. They have taken away from so many girls' lives. I'll be damned if they take me. It is such bullshit. I am pissed off and my distorted thinking is just as much a part of the addictive obsession. The majority of girls do not take their dysfunctional eating or thinking to the point of physically needing to seek professional help. However, I don't believe you have to take it to an extreme to address the issue. I can't even begin to count all the girls and women who in some way allow food, weight, or their body image to control their lives or turn to food for control. I could bet my life that every woman at some point has thought, "If I could just get my weight under control I would be so much happier and my life would be so much better." They believe that having a perfect body and good eating habits are directly correlated to being happy.

Nothing bothers me more than the media sensationalizing eating disorders. Their ignorant and futile attempt to simplify the disease and fascinate their readers' and viewers' "inquiring minds" rarely addresses more than the shock-value elements and the extreme cases, making eating disorders all the more easily dismissable and removed. This is not some rare disorder. I bet one in two women on a regular basis worries about gaining weight and is always in touch with the scale's fluctuating numbers and with the way their clothes fit. I can't remember the last time I was around a group of women when food and weight were not one of the major topics discussed. Women don't make food choices by desire or taste but by the weight and calories attached to each bite. These women are not ignorant about what goes in their mouth and how it will affect their bodies. It's true some may care one day and not the next, but the majority of women are terrified of how an increase in their size or shape will affect the grand scheme of life as they know it or hope to experience it.

As to what makes one woman take her preoccupation too far, the reasons vary. Many women don't even realize they have an attachment to food. Nor do they feel their attitudes are different from any of their friends, so they feel they must be fine. They believe they have no need to think there could be something better than living with obsessive thoughts and anxiety over their bodies.

I found peace for a while in my obsession. Eating disorders are not as bizarre, abstract, or distant as people would like to think. I am not saying that most women are on the verge of an eating disorder. Nor am I trying to make myself feel better through generalizing my problem. But I do think that many women turn to food, weight, and exercise as a means of coping with life and its struggles. I believe we are doing ourselves a disservice by keeping this taboo disease at arm's length. For whatever reason, it took going into treatment to realize that an obsessive addiction with food and my body had taken control of me and would not take me where I wanted to go.

This is not that crazy when you stop to think about it. Behind all the symptoms, rituals, and darkness is the woman you know and love who is scared to death and feels desperately alone in her responsibility to make her life and the lives of others stay on course. She is not crazy nor is she a freak. Her actions may seem crazy and bizarre, but she is not. She is scared. I never thrived by being kept at arm's distance. I needed to know I was loved and that the concerns of my family and friends were out of love. I wanted to hear I was loved because I began to believe there was nothing there to love. From my perspective I was failing at my mission, which was making other people as happy as I could and doing everything orderly and perfectly. My inability to fulfill my ideals was fair grounds for others not to love me or accept me. In their eyes I could see the freak they thought I was. People no longer related to Chelsea but to the symptoms of the disease.

Just because I was diagnosed with an eating disorder does not mean I am not separated from those with milder forms. I was there once also. I don't think eating disorders are as bizarre or as identifiable as the media has portrayed them to be. I am not a victim of this disease or the stigma attached to it.

For me the eating disorders and the preoccupation with food were symptoms of a much deeper struggle with the emotions, feelings, circumstances, and memories that I did not know how to cope with. And at that time I did not have the skills to work through them. It started off so innocently. I simply wanted to lose weight, wanting to feel and look better. For whatever reason I began to feel better and found comfort in my success. It was a healthy and rewarding distraction. Without consciously realizing it, I began to rest in the knowledge that anytime I needed to get away, think about something else, relieve stress, or find immediate gratification, I knew how to achieve it. It was no big deal, not life-threatening; in fact I was much healthier.

Slowly my new lifestyle took me away from almost any upset, fixing that which I didn't know was even bothering me or stirring within me. "Too much of a good thing is not good." My belief that I had control grew increasingly further from the truth. Unconsciously I could depend on my body to make them okay and make the immediate context of my world rational and orderly. When everything else was going wrong I knew how to make it right, make it smooth. I became dependent and addicted to removing myself from the pain I was too afraid to face. Increasingly my need to maintain the level of relief led me to choose purging and starving to cope with my inability to achieve my high ideals. All the while I was running further from the truth in my life. The more fixated and preoccupied I became, the more sense my thoughts and choices made. The mutilating and destroying of my body felt so fitting. My puerile experience with sexual abuse made the rituals seem okay, even appropriate to the way the darkness felt inside. I simply could not see, feel, or believe what everyone else saw the outside to be. Even in my own reality I thought I was lying. My eating disorder was the way I unconsciously chose to manifest and release my pain. The pain could have been everyday stress or just life struggles no different than those of any other human.

I needed to hear that you cared, that you were scared, and that your greatest fear was losing me. Seeing you cry was okay. Just because I knew no other way to ask for help didn't mean that you couldn't. So many times I wondered if you noticed and if you were scared. I wondered how long I would be like this and how long we would pretend it would go away. I never expected you to fix it. In fact, your efforts only made it worse. The best thing you did for me was to take care of you and show me you wanted more for your life than feeding my addiction and watching it grow. I can't imagine how difficult it must have been trying to arrange and articulate the words just right. The order didn't matter, but the love did, the acknowledgment and confessions of truth did. I am sorry, I am so sorry. Looking back now I loathe thinking of the pain and anguish I caused you all. I hate that I was the source of so much fear and pain in your lives. I know I took it too far, but I have come to a place where I can be grateful for my eating disorder. Please know I never did it to make you suffer. If I had never gone through this, my life would not be as rich or as real, nor would I be this strong. I am passionately grateful I do not live with the secrets and the pain I once did. Most of it you didn't know was there. I have been given the most amazing friends and the most supportive and real family imaginable, all of whom exemplified unconditional love. This was a new path for all of us and none of us did it perfectly, but we obviously did something right. I must say it started with God.

CO⁀CO

Boy, this is really hard for me. I am trying so hard to please people that I don't even have a clue what I myself really want. I have the hardest time knowing what to do with choices because I don't want to let anyone down or disappoint anyone. I have these ideals in my mind of what a typical college student does and if I don't meet those expectations then I feel as though I have failed or that I am not doing well in recovery. I like to know where I am and what to expect. I like to feel safe.

But then I start getting into other's perceptions of my life and their judgments. I try to figure out what I could do better or what they think I should be doing. My life will never be perfect. I guess it really is a process and learning acceptance of the unpredictable present moment. I hate it. I am walking around clueless as to what to do or say or what hurts. I thought recovery would be different, or maybe I thought I would be different in recovery, that I would be the exception to the norm. I am not. I am human and trying to live and learn the stuff I missed somewhere along the way. I am so caught up in what I am not that I am not accepting what I am and what I am becoming. I am not perfect and I don't have the keys to my life. I guess I am struggling the best I can.

◯◯

I can't and won't live the lies I hear whenever I start to
focus on my body. The lies are a gift, not my enemy but a red
flag that in some way signals other stuff is going on, not what I
feel is going on.

◯◯

I swear I have put on ten pounds. Fine. Fat is not a feeling, but I sure as hell feel something. If I eat one thing more
than what my mind has set as the standard before I eat, I think
it's all over. My body is going to blow up. I went to this mixer
last night and it was fine for awhile, but then I had enough. I
went home so upset with myself because if I was normal I would
have stayed there all night and been drunk with all my friends.
So I chose to stare at myself in the mirror, trying to see how my
body had drastically changed in the course of a few hours. I
started to look at the old thin pictures and I liked what I saw. I
still think that is attractive. It is really horrible looking. What is
up? Why am I buying into this? I have some choices. I can stand
in front of this mirror and make myself feel like hell for eating
three cookies or I can walk away and go read some healthy-
thinking stuff. I can tell myself it is okay and that I may not love
every party I go to but that I can be grateful that I know what
I like and don't like. My futile attempt to control life and my
extreme thinking leave no room for choices. When I think that
things are either right or wrong, like that I can either throw up
or be fat, I miss the middle ground. I don't give the shadows
due credit. The rest of the world does not place such rigid ultimatums on itself. I don't have to choose to see just the black
and white. I can choose to see in between.

I want to live my life, not fear it. I want to stop living out
my nightmare of a life and stop living as a stranger to myself. It
is so scary going through my day, every day being with someone I never wanted to encounter who in some bizarre way

knows they know everything about me but who I usually can't even begin to figure out. When I see her in the mirror, she is just as scared of me and of who I am capable of becoming—and even more of what I am capable of conquering. But when I don't recognize Chelsea, I am terrified, because I never know what will be thrown my way.

⚬⚬

I probably get weirded out once a day, at least I have for the past two days. It sucks. I get so fearful and I'm sure nothing is going to work out. I've been back in Fort Worth for two weeks. I didn't have time to even breathe before I had to start the fall semester at TCU. This ceramics class I'm taking has me all worked up. I am convinced I won't get it all done. Then I get upset with myself for not devoting enough time to school stuff. I want so badly to make a 3.0 so I will have options. Maybe I am expecting a lot to think that by the end of my first semester of college I will know how to study, and to manage my time, my recovery, my money, and just being away from home.

⚬⚬

I will catch myself looking at other girls' bodies to see whether I am okay. For example, I might look at a girl in class and see how she acts with her body. I wonder what she thinks about it and what she tells herself about her body. I watch how she lives in her body and wonder if she is happy or sad. I wonder what she feels like living in that body shape. I will see a girl and think she is cute and has a good figure. I can see that her size is not that different from mine. She looks happy. Maybe I am okay too. When I was working so hard at becoming emaciated, I never thought about those things. I knew what I wanted and liked the results I was getting. Despite the fact that I always fell short of how I wanted to look, I was defining my own self-image, adhering to my high ideal, and holding my head high. I couldn't compare myself to anything but pictures in magazines because that was the only way to be. I never realized how obsessed I was with pictures of models until I wrote this paper for English. I liked one part that I wrote. I don't remember exactly how it went, but I based it on an article in Bazaar magazine entitled, "Body of Evidence." My body was evidence that I was dying.

∽✿∾

I heard that when you don't feel something (that you want to feel), you act as if it were so.

∽✿∾

My back is killing me. That usually means something is going on. I will never have a perfect body (as if I know what one is). I have this illusion that a perfect body will give me power and control over my life. It does not take a genius to know that men usually don't like women who are heavy, so I guess having a good body means having more control over men. I don't know a guy who would not drop his life for Cindy Crawford. I remember telling Dr. Tant something to that effect. She responded with, "How do you feel about guys having sex with you in their minds?" I responded with the obvious, "No, I don't want that, and I sure as hell did not think that's what would happen if I had a perfect body." Maybe it is easy for me to believe that others criticize my body because I do. Maybe it has more to do with the way I see myself than with the way I assume they see me. I believe with all my heart that a person who has high self-esteem, knows herself within, and believes in herself is the most beautiful gift to the world and to her own life. These are the people who glow when you see them. They

DIARY OF AN EATING DISORDER

are so full of life. They have found joy in just being. I can't get enough of those people.

∽∽∽

Maybe this is part of God's plan. I am failing. I feel like my life is crazy. I don't know how to function now that my means of coping has been stripped. I don't know how to handle much. I am scared. I don't know how to take care of myself. The way I took care of myself before almost killed me. Feeling lost and confused is part of growing up, and my expectation to have a happy-go-lucky life sets me up to be a failure. I need help. I can't do it alone. I don't know what that means, but I do need help. I am scared, I don't want to commit myself to other obligations and be expected to be in some other place.

∽∽∽

Day in and day out I may not throw up, but I restrict a little. I would like to restrict what I eat a little more. I turn to food for security and happiness. I am still addicted and afraid as hell because I don't have a clue how or where to begin with my life. My life? That is so weird. I don't even know whose life I am living. I am not always living mine for sure. I am not what my heart feels. Nor what my soul believes. I am so tired of planning everything I do, making lists, expecting situations to be just the way my mind has painted them, expecting nothing but the best from myself, expecting my role in others lives is to make their lives better. I believe I can at least do my part, and my part is to make them happy.

∽∽∽

Well look at today! It is ten months since Remuda. AWE-SOME! I have been working some stuff out in my head. I think I have been expecting a lot from myself considering I have not been in recovery that long. Thinking that I would come out of Remuda and just soar with flying colors of success is not realistic, nor is my condemnation of not meeting the high standards helpful.

These past few days I have been stricken with fear, fear that my body is changing and going to pot. It is as though I woke up and fear had taken charge. It really sucks. I defiantly have started lying and telling myself that I am in charge. What a joke! I have been feeling that I will have to go away to find happiness, but that doesn't seem right either. I have myself wherever the location is and that is where I should look. I want an identity so badly. I hear in my head what I think Mom would say it should be or what the world would say it should be. It clouds my own thoughts and leaves me more confused than when I initially posed the simple question to myself. I will question if I should brush my teeth before or after I take my shower knowing there is a better and more efficient choice. I want to have something to call my own that I will know myself by and others will say, "Oh, that is so Chelsea." I would love to be an incredible athlete. I imagine myself doing awesome things like all these back flips and layouts, all of which come so naturally, or being able to run so fast that I would be the next Jackie Joyner-Kersey.

∽∾

Today was living hell. I have just arrived in LA to visit my dad. That in itself is not the hell. Rather it was the anxiety the visit created. I stopped at nothing. All the negative, self-defeating thoughts I could possibly have rang true today. This day last year was very different. I had my head in a toilet. I am grateful I didn't even think about that being one of my options today. I am fighting not to drink this laxative tea my dad has, the same stuff I drank when I was actively into my disease. I just keep telling myself, "Fake it till you make it." Fake all the things

I know to be true in recovery until the feelings match the truth. It was all I could do to recall the way I was before I got in the plane. I pictured myself walking the path I knew was the one I must walk to continue in recovery, to continue to live.

Visiting here has never been easy. This time is no exception. Dad and Jude are separated. I had been praying really hard for them to work things out, but I guess the separation is good if they feel it to be necessary. I have never spent any amount of time alone with my dad, so I had mixed feelings about Jude's absence. Dad and I went to my favorite restaurant. I hope we never go again. Despite my desire and our agreement for him not to drink in my presence, he ordered a bottle of wine, of which I had none. As the appetizers came, the conversation seemed to flow. I volunteered information about my life (he doesn't have a clue what to ask). We talked relatively well, but dinner seemed to take forever. I became increasingly angry and anxious over the long wait. By the time dinner came, I was so angry I had no appetite left. In the midst of my dad philosophizing about my life (the one he doesn't know), I glanced down and realized that my anger had nothing to do with the belated arrival of food but with the bottle of wine he had polished off. I was so disgusted.

His first swallow of wine seemed to start his tongue. With every word that followed my realization I just wanted to scream and say, "Shut the fuck up. You don't know jack about my life and for that matter about me. What gives you the nerve to ramble and hypothesize about the direction in which my life is going?" I just became so disgusted that my life was being planned and treated so casually by this man who was drunk and totally unaware. The lump in my stomach grew. I didn't have to be a silent victim nor a silent but consenting supporter of his unrecognized alcoholism. I shut down and ate my food. I just kept saying to myself, "I'll be damned if I let him get in the way of my recovery."

I knew that I did have choices—I could leave or tell him how I felt. In retrospect I would have. I would have told him again, like a broken record, and then in his belittling way he would have told me I was making a big deal out of nothing and that my mom put these ideas in my head. I just hate more than anything that when the waiter asks what we want to drink he looks at me as though I am an overprotective parent or insane girl. Discounting all prior conversations, Dad asks my permission in a condescending tone if it would bother me for him to have a drink. (Sometimes he must not be in the mood to mess with the sarcasm or the unspoken messages and he orders a nonalcoholic drink.) I just felt so angry every time he had a sip. It was as though his act was saying, fuck you, fuck your feeling, fuck our time together, and fuck taking the time to get to know a little bit about your life. I can't help but think, "Isn't it the least you could do not to drink so you could remember one thing I tell you?"

Why I expect it to be different I don't know. Maybe I am still living out the way I imagined you all those years you were gone. You didn't leave much to go on so my childhood fantasy was far better than anything like the reality of our relationship. No matter how hard I wish this weren't so, it still is. But I did what I had to and I am okay. Thank God I realized it wasn't me and that I never had to be in this situation again.

∞∞

Change is a true blessing from God. I didn't even write these past few days. I wanted to wait until I had some idea of what was going on inside. Perhaps the pain was so great I just held it in. I now know where some of this present sadness is coming from. About a week ago my grandmother called me and asked if I would come over because she needed to talk with me. I thought it strange to begin with, but when I got to her house I was all the more troubled.

"Chelsea, I wanted to talk to you about going to Trisha's wedding." My heart sank as her downhearted eyes revealed her fear of my disappointing her. "I know what you think happened when you were little, but I think it wasn't like you thought. It was not that big of a deal." Staring at the speckled linoleum floor, holding my sight on one beige speck hoping the trance could withstand the onslaught of my emotions. I fought to hold back my tears. She continued, while flashes of Trisha touching me flashed in a continuous, nauseating rhythm. I tried to focus but her words were of little weight compared to my memory of the act committed in the room just above my head. "Will you just go to the wedding for me? I don't ask much of you and I just can't bear what her family will think if you do not go. Please don't do this to me. It is so important for me to have you there."

I got up from the kitchen table I had eaten at most of my young life. I had brought much to and taken much from that table. Maybe I was not so crazy never to speak of Trisha touching me. After Michael was so desperately forgotten by all who knew, why should she be dealt with any differently? At four going on five, I instinctively knew her assault would be not only accepted but excused. I protected them from hearing something they could never unhear. It was true. I could see it in her eyes, a comforting lie is preferable to a disturbing truth. My shaming secret boiled inside. I was terrified. The truth has strange qualities. Embracing the memory alone, I came to understand the truth to lie in a nasty, shaming, guilty event. Even though I knew what she did at thirteen was wrong, I chose not to tell.

Something about a girl molesting a girl was so horrible to me. I could see how a guy might, but a girl doing it was just far too humiliating. I don't want to think about her touching me, but I do. The memory is not only shameful but nauseating. I remember Mimi periodically calling upstairs, asking us if we were okay and Trisha saying, "Fine." I never told a soul how she played with my body like a pliable doll. The thing I don't get is that my mom and grandmother never said they didn't believe it—both were so quick to excuse Trisha. It probably happened to her and she didn't know any better they said. How can they seek to understand the source of her motives when they don't fully accept what happened to their own daughter? The sad part is that I moved from knowing the truth and understanding the wrong in my gross, impure feelings to dismissing her impact on my life. My family now knows what took me thirteen years of silence to reveal. I can't conceive of my mother's reality, seeing Trisha's mother and having to pretend that nothing happened. Maybe this is my weakness, too. By not confronting Trisha and her family, I too, continue the secret. Still, knowing all you know now, how can you talk as though it never happened? In your mind it keeps the waters smooth. Tell me this: Would you tell your blond, curly headed four-year-old baby that it was okay Trisha touched her and taught her to feel things she never needed to know simply because it probably happened to Trisha? Besides, you say, she is so young and her mother is your friend. You might as well have said these things, because you now know all that I have known this secret to be, and nothing's changed.

So much had been brought to that table, so many secrets that were never wanted, and never allowed to breathe. But this addition felt like the weight of the world to me. By asking me to celebrate this woman's wedding, to dress up and pretend that I had these joyous and celebratory feelings toward her felt like selling my soul—like lying, deceiving what I loved despite what she stole. My grandmother was telling me that this horrible memory I've yet to shed wasn't real, much less spoken of—that it didn't really happen. Then in pure desperation she attempted to guilt me into pretending everything was okay.

The hard part is that my grandmother is as close to me as

my mother. She raised and loved me with the closest thing to unconditional love that I had known. I did not want to make this choice. I knew by not going I would bring her shame and embarrassment. By going I would continue to live in my darkest secret, carrying on its power over me. I couldn't believe how desperate she was to sell out to appearance over truth and morality. Her generalization rearing broke all ties of defense and honesty. I could never hold her manipulative tactics against her. I don't blame her for not wanting to believe I was molested in her own home. I had held on to the secret since that day when I was four and Trisha's actions changed the course of my life forever. I struggled to let go of my grandmother's desire for my attendance and participation in the celebration. I love her more than anything, but now I could do something about my pain by not willingly selling myself out. I had to live the truth. I had to tell her no.

Her heartbroken voice left me empty and so guilty. She was not happy with me. It just seems like this time I can do something. I can say no by not going. I know she has not forgotten that day. It would suck for her as well. One thing is for sure, I didn't give in to my eating disorder. The thinking was the most painful part. It would have been so easy to succumb to the call of the cycle. "My mind is a scary place to go all alone." Thank you Lord.

God, if you want me to go and face Trisha and Michael someday please give me the strength and opportunity to do so.

∽∾

I had the biggest blast. Our formal was last night and I asked this guy who I sort of know. We had a great time together. Chad was so nice, very funny, handsome, and great to dance with. I can't believe that we have been going to the same school all semester and not until now did we meet. We had so much fun together. He makes me laugh so hard and is very charming.

Knowing that Chad is aware that I was in a treatment center for an eating disorder is weird, especially since we have never
discussed it. I do not like him knowing an intimate part of my
life told by someone else. Elizabeth and I had gone over to the
guys' dorm and had planned for her to leave Chad's room so I
could talk to him about my eating disorder and lay it out on the
line. I couldn't stand not addressing it any longer. I wanted him
to know the truth from me. The whole opening was embar-
rassing. I am sure it was obvious Elizabeth didn't really need to
visit Mark's room on the second floor. A lot of small talk was
taking place, but I had another agenda planned. "Chad I know
you already know this about me, but I feel a need to tell you
from my perspective about my eating disorder and recovery."
He seemed as surprised at my abrupt opening as I did. Still,
without hesitation he said, "Yes, I do know about you having
an eating disorder, and I was trying to figure out a good way to
bring it up." I continued, telling him the highlights of the past
few years, consciously editing the unsafe or shaming periods.
He was very inquisitive and complimentary of my success. I
really enjoyed talking to Chad. We had a great conversation.
His sister has an eating disorder, so he had some knowledge
about them. I really admired his faith in God to take care of her
and his family. I think it takes a lot of guts for a guy to express
his feelings about God, especially to a girl he hardly knows. I am
so grateful to have him as a friend. He is really a kind and compassionate person. He is such a charmer.

Tuesday was the first meeting of the ABA (Anorexics and
Bulimics Anonymous) group that I have started. It went pretty
well considering the newness and all. Not many showed up. It
was strange holding it in my house, but we already have plans

162

to move to a neutral spot. Lord, I am really praying that you will help bring this group together. I know how desperate we are for a strong recovery group.

◯◯◯

I can't believe that Bret and I are no longer together. I don't know what is changing or what has changed. I can't say where things are going with me now. I am afraid, I don't know why I am confused, and I don't want to lose one of my best friends. He told me that I don't look at him the same way. I couldn't lie; I guess I am easily read. He was right. For once in my life I am allowing myself freedom to do what I want. I am having so much fun dating a guy in college, hanging out with all of his friends, staying out as late as I want on any night I want, and not having to answer to anyone, especially myself. I just don't care. I find myself carelessly letting go and having the time of my life. I am so happy when I am with Chad and his friends. Things couldn't be more perfect. My friends love his and we all have a great time together. Bret's life is so different and I unfairly resent that he can't do the same stuff I can. But he is not supposed to yet. He still has so much to enjoy in high school. And here I am nagging him about something over which he has no control. I wish he would believe me that it was nothing he did. Today I don't know what will happen, nor do I know what the "right" thing is. Lord, I pray for your will to be done.

◯◯◯

For the past two days I have had so much fun. I felt so much relief when I finished finals. I went to the Dave Matthews concert with Chad. I didn't get home till 5:00 in the morning. Then last night we went to hear Robert E. Lee, a blues singer. The moment we walked in the door he set my purse down, and we danced the rest of the night to whatever was playing. He is so much fun because he doesn't care about anything. He just wants to have fun. Chad helps me see how much there is to celebrate in life. I hated for the night to end. We danced and laughed forever. We stayed out till 4:30. He left the next morning to go back home.

∞∞

Well I really don't want to write at all, but I don't want to start believing that I am in charge of my life. Things have been great lately. I can't stop thinking about how much fun I had with Chad. He called and invited Elizabeth and me to come down to Austin to celebrate New Year's with him and all of his friends. Elizabeth just has to go. I will die if I miss this. I think I will have the time of my life.

∞∞

As I walked into aerobics for the first time since Remuda I thought some earth-shattering thing would occur. Maybe God's voice over the p.a. system: "Chelsea, stop. Go home. You shall not do this. Aerobics is not where I want you to be." I was shocked that I didn't have some sign saying, "No Chelsea, this is not a good choice for your recovery." Maybe I got a little anxious, like I would freak out, but I was fine and took it really slow. I didn't think about much. It was really kind of nice. I just went very slow. I made a conscious effort to not look in the mirrors. That is hard when the walls are covered with them.

∞∞

Today seems more crippling than normal. I have become focused on my food intake and body's appearance. The reasons I am obsessing again are still left to be told. I am so excited Chad has invited Elizabeth and me to come to Austin for New

Year's and stay at his house. I am sort of nervous about staying at his house and meeting his family. It's not like we are dating at all, but I have heard so many wonderful things about his family. I know I will like them. Everyone says how nice and beautiful his mom and sister are. I feel anxious, excited, and nervous. They probably think it is strange to have these two girls coming to stay at their house. I will have to give it to you, Lord. Just help me be myself and be calm.

I must have been ten or eleven before I would finally admit to myself that what my brothers had told me about Santa was true. Since then the whole Christmas thing has gone downhill. Being the youngest, I was always the most enthusiastic and excited to get presents. As I got older I still wanted to give everyone the joy of watching me get so enamored by all the gifts I received. I felt it was my role, my contribution to Christmas morning. It began to feel like a production. At sixteen the insanity hit. I was in midsprint to leap into my parents' embrace, praising them for the Franklin Word Speller. Then I thought, "What the hell am I doing?" What a fool I feel like and must look like, not to mention how completely irrational I was being. I had just received a word speller. I felt so damn guilty because what had once come so naturally wasn't that natural anymore. The next year I went to the opposite extreme. I hardly said two words, which of course made me look like the biggest brat. So this year I've started thinking about a new way to approach Christmas. There is always such a buildup, and then it is all over and everyone feels sort of let down. Moreover the expectations I put on myself to act a certain way are ridiculous. I am not going to take my family's Christmas joy on as my responsibility. I know they don't even want me to do that. When I wake on Christmas morning, I will know that the gifts of this world will always be a letdown. Never will they measure up to the most perfect gift we all receive, Jesus. I will focus on the real reason we are all together celebrating and knowing the rest is just an added bonus. Since my family is as good as they come, being with them alone is a wonderful celebration. As for the Oscar-winning performance, I will give someone else the privilege of winning, because I have been the reigning champ far too long.

∞∞

So, so much has happened. This New Year's Eve was the best of my life. I haven't felt this strong or at peace in a long, long time. The three nights I spent at Chad's house were perfect. His sister, mom, and the whole family were extremely welcoming and so sweet to Elizabeth and me.

Chad was so cute about New Year's. He obviously worked very hard to plan everything out. The night started with a Mexican dinner at his house, and all of his friends came over to eat. He had made reservations at this really cool jazz club. When we danced together, I felt like a princess, just floating on air. Never could I have dreamt of a better night. The closer midnight got, the more I wanted it to hurry. I have never wanted to start a new year more. In the back of my mind I knew they must be yelling Happy New Year! I was so lost in our first kiss, all I consciously knew was that I wanted time to stop. It was like a dream. I was having the time of my life with all these fun people, with this great guy, and our first kiss on the new year. We danced so much. Chad is so much fun. I think it is great how he couldn't care less what he looks like or what people think. I had forgotten how much I love to laugh and make others laugh. I think it is exciting to be unsure where things stand between us or what will happen. He's told me already that he likes me, but maybe he means it in a not-so-big-deal way. The last thing I want is another relationship. I like to think about him, but the best part is that I love myself when I am around him and am proud to be who I am. I never thought about that being so important until I experienced it. I would have it no other way now.

One lesson I learned through dating Bret and working my recovery is prayer. Praying for God to fix me and make things or me better was praying for my will, not God's will. I trust you, God, that you know best, so I will try my best to let go and go with the flow. I think it is so important for me to trust what I know, not what I think I know, like the "right" solution or what "should" be happening in my life. I am just so glad to know Chad. He will be a great friend. He is one of the coolest guys I have met.

I've had the best time in the world. His family is so great and I have loved meeting all of his friends. I can hardly believe that I ever struggled with food. It's like I am having too much fun to think about anything that meaningless. I eat spontaneously; I eat what I am given. I feel as if I couldn't be any happier with my life. I have this awesome sense of acceptance—acceptance of my surroundings and, most of all, of myself and the life I have.

∞∞

I am not able to sleep. My dad is having major financial problems, so the check he promised me would not clear for tuition. I am scared. Nothing I do makes much difference. Tonight we have another ABA meeting. There are some new girls coming and we have moved the location. I have so much to be thankful for in my recovery. I was shocked when a woman came up to me in Alanon and asked me to come and speak to an Alateen group. I am really excited. All this stuff that has been going on has left little time for me to worry about my body.

Lord I don't know how school will get paid for, but my dad has never been able to handle money well and I sure will not be the one to change him. All I know to do is pray for him and let you help him, Lord. I need to know how to handle my feelings about his inconsistency in sending my allowance on time or at all, and the possibility that I won't be able to go to school next semester because he has not paid. I would pay if I could, but right now, I can't. It is just hard when I see how they live: a beautiful house, the new BMW and new Cherokee they drive. He always has some excuse as to why or how he has what he has, but always closes with, "Chelsea, your education comes first. It is the most important thing in my life." Well, I want to say that's pretty sad if the most important thing to you is falling through, but let me guess: It's not your fault.

All this stuff with my dad has helped me see that I do enable him. I am really afraid that if I start yelling, he will up and leave me. I've always been the sweet one, the one who hasn't been a problem or the source of any conflict. Now I have this money issue, and I don't know how to deal with it. I feel so guilty that most of my calls are reminding him my allowance is late or that he needs to pay for school. Wishing our relationship to be different holds little weight in face of the reality. I try so hard to arrange the words just right, hoping something will change. Even though he is the adult, I've always viewed our relationship as my responsibility and my downfall.

⟡

Chad came back to school early. We went out and had a great time. Last night everything changed. Our date was ending like most, sitting, talking, and making each other laugh. We started talking about our past relationships, then he expressed how much he enjoyed being with me and that it would bother him if I had a date with another guy. Of course I was loving this.

Here is Chad, as charming and wonderful as ever, telling me he would hate it if I dated anyone else. Somewhere between my coy giggling and wallowing in his words of adoration, Chad and I were exclusively dating each other. As I kissed him good night, it was all I could do to contain myself.

Then, as quickly as the joy had come, the reality set in. I had relinquished all the freedom of my newly acquired lifestyle. Yes, I do like Chad, but I really hadn't intended for this to happen so fast. I was just getting into this whole dating thing. I liked the way things were. There was a mystery and an attraction to the unspoken feelings, wondering whether I liked him and he liked me. I love the freedom and I had just stopped dating Bret. I don't know what to do. I didn't want anything serious. Yuck, I feel trapped. I like him, but it has happened way too fast. This makes me sick. I don't want to start playing games because of my inability to express my feelings. (I usually do, which screws things up more.) I am glad that I am easygoing about this. It feels good not to have such intense feelings or a need to act on my immediate emotions. I am not in middle school. I can't turn around and tell him that I want to break up or get Lauren to do it for me.

⋘⋙

Last night Chad and I had a good long talk. I sort of broke down. He, of course, knows about my eating disorder. I think it is both good and bad that he knows about the mess this disease creates. I put so much pressure on myself to figure out what everyone needs me to be and arrogantly take sole responsibility for any mood that is not happy, joyous, and free. I also assume that the way I am couldn't possibly be right. But what I needed to tell him (for myself) was that I had to stop trying to be so perfect and that I am going to screw up. I don't know how to be a perfect girlfriend, even though I try.

Of course he had no idea that I was trying to be. Unless you are a perfectionist or a very driven person, it's hard to imagine the intensity with which every situation is confronted. It must seem crazy to someone who is not driven by the desire to do everything right. It's not like I am trying to be this way. It just seems to me that for my life to function, I have to run at 110 mph all the time. When I stop to think about my need for the sock drawer to be neatly organized or the bed to be made just right, it is directly related to the order and cohesion with which my life will run. I have found by not beating up on myself, like for not making my bed one day, I let go of my intense drive and see that everything is okay without the bed being perfect.

∽∾

Today in my Alanon meeting I heard a lot of good stuff. There is a difference between love-based and fear-based feelings and the choices you make as a result. New beginnings are about doing things differently. "Do the next right thing"—the one lesson that really fits. When I feel out of control with my own life I tend to focus on controlling myself and, most of all, others. When controlling others doesn't work, my distorted thoughts and eating-disorder symptoms start up big time. When I look to others to fill the emptiness inside myself, I have this idea that if they treated me in just such a way or said just the right things, then they could fix me. They never do, of course, and I always end up worse off because of my expectations. It is hard to just sit in the pain, but sometimes that's all I can do. I have this belief that I can get Chad to treat me all the time like he does when he is in a great mood. If I am funny, charming, or cute enough, I feel sure he will treat me the way I love to be treated. If he doesn't, I assume it is my shortcoming. How can I think that way? It's not always in relation to me. I am not always in it. Chad's mood probably has nothing to do with me and I don't have the right to assume it does. It is a sad lie to think I am less if I fail at getting him to be wonderful. I must admit it pisses me off that I can't, that I am not good enough to have that ability. At least I am starting to believe that I can't, and at least I am aware. It is sad that I will really believe that someone else's bad mood or complacency is my fault and that when I can't change it I will think they must not like me. No wonder I have been using body as a distraction to all this crap I tell myself. This pressure is absurd.

Lord, help me see that not everything is my fault and that I cannot fix other people. I turn my will and life over to you.

∞∞

I feel confused, overwhelmed, and uncertain. My dad and I have not talked in a long time. I know he is there, but he feels so far away.

I feel that my life is my responsibility—I mean, to make it all happen, to figure everything out. I don't know what is going on inside. I feel so confused. I am in fear of the future. Is God punishing me or trying to tell me something? I am so afraid I have done something to turn God away. I don't think he can hear me. I don't get it. What am I not doing that I should be? I want to eat and exercise. I have thought about food a lot. I am trying so hard to figure out the perfect schedule. In my mind it's like putting a perfect little puzzle together. I love the challenge of organizing, and if it all falls into place, I win. All my thoughts, actions, and decisions are such a big deal. George (in Alanon) always says there are not big deals. I am just going to assume that God not being here has more to do with me than with him. So we need to talk. I need to find you in me, God, because I know you are there.

☜☞

John Holt and John have been the best brothers in the world. They used to tell me that the first time I had a date they were going to stand on the roof and pee on the guy as he came to the door to pick me up. And then they would take it so far as to say that I couldn't date, because there would never be a guy who could get their approval. When the time came, they didn't go so far as to urinate on him, but they did make it very clear that no guy would ever be good enough for their little sister. I loved their overprotective mentality, but I have always been terrified of letting them meet any guy I date. I cringe with embarrassment, because I know this poor guy is getting grilled in the most inconspicuous ways. One wrong comment from my date and I won't hear the end of it, but it will see the end of him. The good part is that they have protected me from making some dumb mistakes. They taught me about guys' manipulative tactics and how at my age they are full of BS for the most part. Their loving me and protecting me helped me believe I had something special and that I never had to settle.

Bringing Chad to meet the dynamic duo had a different feel to it than with any guy before. I decided that I didn't care how they felt about Chad, nor did I care what they had to say. I didn't want to hear a word about it. I will admit that I was surprised when I saw Chad and John Holt having a Samuel Smith Oatmeal Ale together and smoking cigars. My instinct was right that Chad could hold his own with my brothers. I wasn't so sure whether I liked it or not.

The Trash Disco Party itself was great. I danced forever as always and I acted crazier than most of the people there, and would you believe I had nothing to drink? Dancing really keeps me close to my heart. I have never been unhappy while dancing. Lately I am reminded of the lack of control I have over my eating disorder and that I just have to go for it. It has been fun.

ᏟᏃᏟᏃ

It's really cool to think that one year ago was my first day at Remuda. My life is so incredible now. I can't even begin to explain how I love my life, and it is a life I didn't know I could love. Yes, it is hard, and most of the time all I write about are the bad or really difficult times. I can honestly say that I have grown thankful for my eating disorder. The eating disorder is not the tragedy but rather the messes that lie beneath the surface are. For me the eating disorder was the catalyst to understanding the darkness in my life, my relationship with and faith in God, my family, and believing in an authentic self. All of my relationships and my sense of being are so different and so much better than I could have imagined possible.

Things have been up and down this whole week, but yesterday and today have been great. I had the best time with Chad and John Holt last night. We all went out together. Both of them are so calm and laid back, and they completely take care of themselves. They have helped me learn to enjoy silence, and not to have this anxious need to fill every moment with talk. I realize that it is okay not to speak when nothing needs to be said. I love my brother more than anything. I wish I could be more like him. He is so smart, open-minded, honest, real, truthful, and compassionate, and he is the funniest person on earth. He loves me so much, and it feels so good to know that with all my heart.

ᏟᏃᏟᏃ

The word addict holds a negative connotation. I hear a choice in its definition. I see a person I would never want to be. I would, if I could, kill that part of me, the part that chose to commit and submit to that little voice and to the darkness within the pain for so many years of my life. It really is a constant struggle to keep my head above water. This is so, so hard. Then I remember God, and I begin to remember to pray for trust, wisdom, and the strength to just wait. No longer do I pray for the cure. I no longer ask why, or how long, although I am still amazed that this was in "the plan." My recovery is truly a war, with a person who was once my best friend. Time will build a retaining wall of confidence in my strength and endurance in recovery. The first year is the hardest, but I am proud of the firm foundation I have laid. I am here to say I made it one year, and I struggled well.

∞∞

I want with all my heart not to be controlled or manipulated by my mind and the food. Running from the truth will never work. One day I won't live with the demon. I don't believe she is forever. Maybe it will click or slowly seep away, dissolve, deteriorate, ultimately to be removed from the cavities of my mind. In my innocence I knew nothing about appearance or what others thought. I just did as I pleased. I had never heard of a calorie or a relationship with food, much less an addiction that feeds off self-hatred. I learned simply to love and live.

# Spring 1995

It has been forever since I wrote you last. There is so much on my mind I could scream. So much I want to say I can't even fathom getting it all down. I got drunk last night and made myself throw up. I am so ashamed. What is going to happen now? I broke my record, I screwed up. I am so messed up. How could I have done this? The more I drank the more my guard fell, and I just didn't care. Then all at once I was consumed with this shame and guilt over what I thought was bad behavior, but here I was having a great time with all my friends. I couldn't let go of how wrong I was to be doing what I was doing. When I got home I ate and then told myself I had really screwed up, and I could not handle that. What I saw to be lack of control and lax attitude would cause me to gain weight and be fat and disgusting. Obviously the food didn't fix the shame. Nor did I make my wrong right. I gave in and threw up. There is no way around it. I did it and I fucked up.

It bothers me that I don't feel guilty as hell today, that I am not belittling myself. I have got to beat myself up. I can't behave that way and let it go. I will do it again. Oh fuck it. All I want is to throw in the towel now. Hide and never come out. I can't fathom trying to go on—taking the next step and facing the reality of my action. I really believed that I had turned my future over to God. I don't get it. Everything seems so right. Why would I go and do that? It just sneaks up on me: Wham! Out of nowhere. I bought into the lies, the freedom, the quick fix. Chad and I are great. I love living with Elizabeth, and all my classes are going well. So am I just crazy? Am I just a screw-up? I am a fat pig. No I am not! I have got to stop telling myself this stuff. Scaring myself into the right feelings and thinking won't work. What the hell is going on inside? All I know now is the symptom. There must be more to this than I can understand now. One thing I know I can do is "eat the next meal," go on, and keep living.

Okay I need to let this crap go—the past and the future. I can get so worked up. Lord, please, with all my heart I am begging you help me live in today and trust you. Please, I am scared about my recovery. I don't expect you to take it away but I need help. All my friends are so great and so supportive, but unless you have lived with this, it's hard to know how to handle it. When I tell my friends that I am struggling, it inevitably changes our relationship. I don't blame them; they care about me and want to help. But when I have told them before, it has become this looming thing between us. I can't blame them for not knowing what to say, but I need them to say something to let me know they heard me. Otherwise my secret just sits on the forefront of our minds, never being verbally addressed, but affecting everything we do. Saying to them, "I want to give up, I don't want to eat, I hate my body!" and expecting them to carry on with things as normal is not realistic. Talking about my pain and anxiety is the best thing. Hell, if all they could say is "Chelsea, I am scared. I want you to be okay, and I am here for you." Anything other than us pretending that nothing was said. The pretending is almost as haunting as the painful secrets.

Real love is encouraging a person's spiritual journey and growth.

I think it has been a saving grace to be able to talk about the stuff that consumes me. Unless I am honest, I go nuts. I feel much better not holding that all inside.

∞∞

What do I lose when I drink? I have no smile inside. The one that might appear is only out of habit. My insides become so dark and heavy. That spark and my spirit become stifled. I can no longer hear the truth. I get into the problem and not the solution. My self-imposed guilt is premeditated. I begin to believe the overwhelming fallacy that everyone else is my responsibility and that I always screw their lives up by not making them happy. I think I need to understand everyone and read his or her mind. It makes me hate myself and feel as though I weigh three hundred pounds. I get sad and lonely. Maybe a more fitting question is, "What does drinking give me?"

Last night was a big deal for me. I ate late-night pizza. I am and have been okay with it, but I can hear that little voice desperately trying to sabotage my tranquillity and acceptance. In the grand scheme of things that pizza will change nothing. It will have no effect on my weight.

∞∞

I have had some realizations about Chad and myself. First, he is a great listener and really helps me separate the lies and see how irrational I can become. I tried to evoke some emotions out of him by not eating. He is not the most expressive person, and without realizing it, I thought that by not eating I could get him to react in some way. I began to realize that in our relationship it is always me who has the problems and he is the one to fix them.

When I tell him my worries he feels useful, like he has a distinct role. Yes, he does make a difference. I think he likes helping me and taking care of my feelings. It's that whole fixing-the-sick-girl thing. But I am not sure I really have an issue every time one is discussed. I see how I feel more cared about and can hear that he cares when I am in need. Our interacting is more personal and substantial. At times Chad can be very aloof and indifferent toward our relationship. When I get his attention with my problem, he treats me much more compassionately. I can see how I feel this duty to tell him a problem no matter how insignificant it might be. Now I am not blaming him for this, but I see my part in it. I have thrown my heartfelt pain out there for him to fix and he does, he rescues me. This is a pattern I really don't want to continue in our relationship. I want more balance, to know more about what goes on with him. I have a ton of friends who know my stuff, all of whom I can talk with, so I am going to use them instead. I need to be separate and have my own life. I don't want to involve him in everything, and I am sure he doesn't want to be. I myself don't like being involved in all that goes on in my life. Why would he?

⟨∞⟩

I am still whining about the same old stuff. It is time to move on. I really have to make a conscious effort not to let other girls' lack of eating and increased drinking get to me. I just keep telling myself that my rules are different. I am not dumb or weird but I am different. Just because I have to eat three meals a day does not make me a pig, even if I have to do it by myself. When they talk about food I try not to let it get to me. I have done my part and told all of them that I have to eat and that talking about fat and calories is really hard for me—especially while we eat. But they still talk about these things, and I have to remember where I have come from and that I have different circumstances. Talking about weight and food is such a part of our everyday lives. We are all so conscious of our bodies and how they are compared to other girls'. Ultimately I must let it go.

⚭

Why do I keep writing? It gets worse before I could even say it's better. I am in Cancun with six of my girl friends. I don't want to feel this bad. I hate many things. This girl named Chris won't shut up about her body and how horrible she will look by the time she gets back. In her whiny voice she says, "I have never missed my exercise program for three days straight! And then there's all this crap I have put into it. I bet I have had sixty fat grams in this one meal."

I ate when I got home and I was not even hungry. It was as though it would satisfy my fear or my feeling alone and nerdy for going home early. I would love to have thrown up. People have told me how blessed and fortunate I am, referring to my recovery. If they only knew how fucked up I was in my head they would have me locked up. Maybe Chris does stuff that reminds me of myself and the way I think sometimes. She puts into words what I fear and what I have lived.

I am carrying around so much stuff that I am sick. I shouldn't say this, but I have been so excited to get home so that I could pick up Chad at the airport. I could hardly contain myself when I saw him get off the plane. It was like the movies. We ran into each other's arms, he picked me up, and I could have kissed him forever. It never crossed my mind that we were in the middle of one of the biggest airports in America. We were so excited to see each other we could hardly talk. I just wanted to freeze the moment and those feeling forever. I was so happy to see his face and his sweet smile. He brought me these beautiful earrings and a great coffee cup. Chad had a great time with his sister. I just need to get out of my head right now, I have so many great things going on. I am not supposed to understand everything nor figure out my every emotion. It is a beautiful day and I'll be damned if I don't live every moment of it.

ᢙᢒᡣᢓ

I am so grateful for Elizabeth's comforting me and supporting me in my recovery. She and Lauren both totally agree that it is important for me to open up to them and not always turn to Chad or keep it inside. She noticed that I was withdrawing into myself and that I was really food-focused. She confronted me, and we talked about it. We decided to make a list of new behaviors and priorities that are more current with my recovery now. I am so glad that she is patient and loves me, even with all my faults and the crazy thinking that she and Lauren struggle to understand. It is great to have someone else to help and share the responsibility. I am just glad she asked because I didn't want to acknowledge that I needed to make some adjustments.

This is my pledge, created by Chelsea and edited by Elizabeth.

My Goals and Things to Remember

1. I am a good person.
2. I love myself.
3. I accept myself where I am.
4. My recovery comes first, and includes
   • meetings
   • counselor appointments
   • daily readings and time with God
   • church
   • patience and trust, one day at a time
   • fun exercise
   • eating what I desire and not what I think is best
5. Stick to my goals.
6. Act, don't react.

7.  Don't pick at my skin or mutilate it.
8.  Don't look at myself critically in the mirror.
9.  Don't throw food away.
10. Don't smash or play with food.
11. Believe the best, and once again, be patient.
12. Talk and express my needs.
13. It is time to get on with my life. Stop dwelling in the problem looking for attention, and envision the positive solution. Imagine myself succeeding.
14. Buy the size clothes I am.
15. Don't be a victim. I am okay.
16. There are NO BIG DEALS.
17. My life is already planned by God. Let it run its course. Let go and let God.
18. Remember everyone who loves me and how much they love me. Envision things they love about me. (In other words, why? They love me because I am who I am.)
19. Don't take responsibility for others.
20. Surrender to reality.

⊙⊙

I'm in pain. I fucking hate this. I am so redundant. My life is not about solutions but about questioning and doubting my every thought and action, not believing a thing I think or feel. It's about wondering whether this is healthy or not, whether my next action will cause me to fall apart, and whether my next move will be right back to Remuda. I sit here and pick at my skin to find some relief. Just like throwing up, it won't fix anything. This is old stuff—feelings, emotions, and behaviors I don't know how to handle. I see the fat or the excess. I want to scream! I push my outer thighs together, making them look like I know they really do, with dimples and all. What the hell is happening? What am I doing that is so wrong? I try so hard. I want to get better so badly. I go to three or four meetings a week, the counselor, and church. I am so fed up with this. I don't get it. All I can say is that I have got to hang on. I am doing my part and there is no quick fix. This just takes time. This is harder than living in my other world.

I don't know why I am so tired, but searching for answers out of fear is not really effective. I want to start living. I wish I could have gone to aerobics yesterday, but it would only prolong the pain. I am a slow learner.

∞∞

Thank you, Lord, for new days and fresh starts. Please help me let go of the past and the future and live in today. I had to call Remuda and tell them I needed a break from all the parents and girls they give my number to for encouragement and reference. It just became too overwhelming and there were too many calls. I feel sort of weird because I think it is my duty to help people, but I need to put my recovery first. I believe in your plan, God, and I am really focusing on loving myself. Our support group has really brought all that home for me. Martha, Cheryl, and I had been praying for it to take off. Now that we meet in Cheryl's office we have a more permanent location. We close every meeting with the Lord's Prayer. I looked at last week's meeting and tears filled my eyes when I saw fifteen girls holding hands, praying and striving for a real and truthful way to live. In that moment I knew God was there smiling, protecting and guiding each one of us in our journey. The group is amazing—a true gift.

∞∞

Chad and I went to the baseball game, and on the way back we got into a discussion. We had not talked in a long time about anything to do with my eating disorder. He asked me about it, and I avoided it for the most part. I didn't want him to focus on me. Finally, I told him some little thing. Now, I have always prided myself on having a keen instinct. But I really wish today that I had never asked Chad a certain question. I already knew the answer, but I think I needed to hear it for myself. So I asked, "Chad, if I don't get over this and put it behind me would you want to stop dating?" His hesitation felt like an eternity. I prefaced the question by asking him to please be honest, and that I truly wanted to know. Collected as always, he said, "Yes I would want to break up if you didn't get better than where you are now." I couldn't say what came after. I had never fought back my emotions and tears as I did at that moment. I just sat there, until he stopped talking, then calmly said, "Thank you for being honest. I am going to go take a shower."

When I got back to the Kappa house I fell into Lauren and Elizabeth's arms. I could hardly get a word out I was crying so hard. All at once I had come up against so many things. This fragile world I held had crumbled, not because Chad would break up with me but because once again I felt the pain of the head-on confrontation with reality. It was the reality that my eating disorder was still very much a part of my life. I had to face the fact that I needed to make a move, I needed to change. At first I hated Chad for saying that. I was so sure he would say no. My gosh, how could he not want to not be with me? Thank God he didn't say no.

Up to this point there had been two major turning points in my recovery and this would have to be one. You see, I couldn't imagine that someone would leave me when I was trying so hard, and I wanted more than anything to put all this behind me. I mean, it's not like I enjoy this life. Who could blame him? Most days I didn't want to even get out of bed for fear of what Chelsea might come up with today. I thought I hid it so well. But I guess I am still not myself or the girl I am wanting to be underneath all this crap. So why would I be so hurt by someone saying he would not want to continue a relationship with a person in a stagnant state of recovery (if there is such a thing)? My first feeling was anger (as was Lauren and Elizabeth's). I wanted to prove to him that I could do it and I would show him how awesome I could be. "You want to see health? Look at me!" The pain and deep crying were not about what Chad had said but the confirmation of what my heart had been telling me for so long.

I know this is not the life I want to live. These days have not been days I want to live, and I am not dissatisfied because of a lack of perfection but because of a lack of truth and a separation from my heart. I don't want this to be my life, but one year and three months into recovery, the reality is that is my life right now and I am fighting for what has always been. Only I can live my recovery, and I will be the one to reap the hard-won and long overdue rewards.

∞∞

I hate my body so much right now. I feel huge. It is hard to believe that fat is not a feeling. I have not been on a scale for almost a year and a half, but I swear I know I weigh 150 pounds. I sure feel like it. I have gained weight, I promise. This sucks so fucking much. I hate it. I almost want to curl up and die.

Outside of today's writing in my journal, I really am so different. I am on top of the world. At least when I'm walking around and doing all that I do, I feel that way. I adore Chad and love all my friends I work my butt off in recovery. When I open this book it's like this stuff just comes out, everything bad and painful. I am glad I have some place safe for it all to go.

I doubt myself all the time. I will be choosing my bagel flavor and think, "No, you shouldn't have that one. This one would be better." I tell myself, "Lauren would do it this way" or, "You should have taken a right there instead of a left." I tell myself that there is always a better way to do everything. I'm always analyzing and second-guessing my choices. When I get around my mom it gets really bad. I still struggle so much with what I imagine she thinks I should or should not be eating. She will come into the kitchen and I will be having a snack and think that she is thinking, "Gosh, Chelsea should not be doing that. All she does is eat." I think a lot of people probably say that to themselves about me. I hate that my friends are indecisive because I always end up coming up with the place we go eat. See, I want to be the easy, giving, laid-back one. I don't want them to think I always have to care where we go. I really don't. They just never will say. Then I tell myself they must think I am controlling.

I have been doing daily meditation but I have not written. It has been a week since my big awareness. This week has been hard but better. I want to get on with things. I have come to realize that my eating disorder is not different from the next person's eating disorder. I am just like them, and it is horrible and so incredibly difficult. I can't go around thinking my addiction is an exception to the rule just because I didn't throw up blood, raid the refrigerator, or starve for three days. I am no different. People ask me whether I still struggle, and I would be lying if I said no. If I didn't struggle I wouldn't be human. Part of where this all began was that I expected superhuman abilities and strength from myself. When stuff bothers me or things are trying in my life, many times I respond through my symptoms. Other times I accept the feelings as just that, and feelings pass. So yes, I do still struggle and think about it. No longer do I say that in shame, because like any person I am learning how to deal with each day as it comes. I now know I was never expected to be superhuman but to be human is enough.

∞∞

I can hardly believe Dr. Don Durham is coming for a convention to educate medical people and therapists here. I get to speak in front of all those people and I am very excited. Girls from the ED group will be there and so will Chad, Lauren, Page, and Elizabeth. I am nervous and excited but definitely thrilled to be on this end.

∞∞

Dr. Don was great! I love him. I know I want to be a speaker. Being in front of all those doctors and therapists was a huge comfort to me in my progress in recovery. I believed in what I was saying and wanted to share with them hope in this disease. I was so grateful to be on this side of the tracks. Really I am so grateful. All my friends were there to watch me speak. They are so supportive. I didn't think I could get up there, but I just kept saying, "be with me Lord, be with me God," over and over until I spoke my first word. I was pumped to get up and tell these parents there is hope, that recovery really can happen. I had forgotten how much pain consumed those watching a loved one slowly self-destruct. You could feel it in the room. The video and lecture were good but not personable or optimistic, perhaps realistic. The opportunity and people fueled me. I couldn't get that microphone in my hands fast enough. I realized how well I am doing and that I am okay. I would be naive to think my perfectionism would not carry over into my recovery. Today I withdrew from my place in the recovery hall of fame and stopped trying to be the best and most perfect. I decided that I am okay. I loved getting be a part of the whole weekend.

⟡

I don't think I know how to love another solution. I turn to myself most of the time. I turn inside, right back where I started. Most of the time I visualize the mistakes I make, and even more, the ones I might make. This negative mental rehearsal doesn't do me any good. I don't think it prepares me to ultimately avoid a mistake. Rather I live out the negative thoughts simply because that is the way I imagined I would do it. When I imagine the failures, I hurt myself and gain nothing. I have nothing to lose and can only gain by visualizing a positive means of handling the situation, believing the good and not the bad. I am capable of so much more and it's amazing that I can accomplish anything, considering how poorly I see myself doing it. I have got to give it a shot.

⟡

I am a little scared. Chad and I got into a fight last night and it seems like we are just not on the same page. I think guys as well as girls make the biggest mistake by staring at someone of the opposite sex and commenting on how "hot" that person is in front of their girlfriend or boyfriend. I think it is the biggest turnoff. You can think it, but save it till you are with your friends.

This bone-thin girl had been strutting around campus, and all the guys caught wind of this new young "thing." That is all he and his friends talked about for three days. They called her the knee-sock girl. "There is something so sexy about a girl wearing black socks above her knees and a short black skirt." I swear if we heard it once this weekend we heard it ten times. I played it off until Chad saw me roll my eyes. He said, "Why don't you wear something like that? You would look cute." I wanted to shove both the bimbo and the knee-sock-lover off a cliff. I was pissed. The nerve of him telling me to dress like this little slut, not to mention the fact she has to have some eating problem. Her thinness is obviously forced. I didn't say all that to him but I tactfully told him how I appreciated that he didn't talk about other girls when I was around (for the most part). I was glad he and his friends were thoroughly enjoying this girl's beauty, but I would rather not hear about it and definitely didn't want him giving me fashion tips based on some anorexic girl.

∞∞

I have been in Austin and in Fredericksburg with Chad and his sister. Elizabeth is living in Fredericksburg for the summer. I am on my way to be a counselor at camp, the same camp where Chad went while growing up. It really was a coincidence that we are going to be counselors together. I almost didn't want to go after I found out he would be there, because I think it will be really hard. I am so excited about getting out of my life, being a friend to all these kids under the age of eleven. I think it will be awesome to teach them and to share about God. So I quickly decided that the experience was more important and that I would have to let the difficult dynamics of our relationship go. I woke up this morning with feelings of fear and aggression. I know this summer will not be easy for my relationship with Chad. I feel this need to claim my independence and my ability to stand on my own. I want to feel joy, the kind I can get only from putting God first in my life. Please, Lord, help me help these kids learn about you. Use me however you need to.

∞∞

I always have a hard time the first few days, and now even weeks, in a new place. I am not surprised by my intense emotions anymore, but it doesn't help that Chad is being such a jerk. I have felt so alone even though I have been with him. I was concerned about our being counselors together, but I've prayed about being here this summer and I feel it is a good choice. I felt so let down and confused by the way Chad is acting. His demeanor of avoidance and aloofness hurts. I hate it. He is not at all like the guy I was dating during school. Chad's aloof and flippant actions really get to me. I hate so much that I can't make him happy and that I can't fix whatever is obviously wrong. I am so upset that I almost threw up. I just have to believe you are in this, God. I have so much stuff I want to say, I don't even know where to start. I need to be mature. I can't cry anymore, and I am not bailing out on these kids because my personal life is all messed up. I will wait it out and trust. My heart feels heavy and alone.

☙❧

Okay, Lord, I am determined to believe in my heart that you brought me to this camp and you are not going to just leave me. I am scared. I've got to be here for the kids and give everything to them. I have so many things in my life to be grateful for. The Hill Country is so beautiful and I really want to grow closer to you through being here, God. This is a new day, a new lesson, and a new chance. Please, heavenly Father, hold my hand so tight, don't let me go. Please let me feel your presence today. I want to take this one moment at a time and above all, trust. I must be okay for these kids.

☙❧

To be perfectly honest I just don't feel an attraction to him. Seeing him act this way I lose respect for him, partially due to his unwillingness to express himself. I cannot and do not want to try to figure this or him out. Caring about Chad as much as I do makes letting go even harder. I find it much easi-

er to care about and be affectionate with someone who recip-
rocates or, even better, initiates. I will, with your strength Lord,
stop trying to read his mind, figure him out, and control our
situation with new actions and new things to say. You are the
only one I can talk to here. Everyone is one of Chad's great
friends and I am "Chad's girlfriend." I believe if I am smart
enough, cute enough, and charming enough I can make him
come out of this. That simply is not so. I don't know what is
right for him, and I question if he even knows right now. I am
here at camp for you, Lord. Help me keep that first.

◌⌒◌

Dear Lord, there are so many things I want fixed and
changed inside me to make things feel okay. Maybe that's just
it. If our relationship is about you and because of you (which I
believe) then it makes sense to let you steer me. "Let go and let
God." This is bigger than I am. I need the tools today to do my
job and help these kids. I will take this one day at a time, take
care of myself, act and not react, and remember my sole purpose. Let the other rest in your most precious hands. While I
sleep, Lord, fill my heart with your love and strength. Don't
leave me.

◌⌒◌

I have prayed on the run and prayed out of fear, and now
I must be still. My true pain is fear, a fear of not being needed
or maybe of being alone. I can hear the fear in my words, I
know my fear in my thoughts, and I can see the fear in my body.
No matter how fast I run it is always faster. For a moment I forget to look. I think I have lost it, but then it all comes back in
my face this time twofold. I am hoping I will acknowledge how
much I am really hurting. I don't know what I need to do, but
I know that taking care of myself and staying in the moment is

the best thing I can do. When I write I really live with the feelings I ball up inside. They never are as bad as I think, but this time I am going to just sit with them and experience what fear and being alone are really like for me.

∞∞∞

Dear God,

Well, I didn't sleep well. That's why I am up at 5:30 in the morning. I am scared, Lord. I haven't been praying as I had hoped I would, especially about camp. I go back in three days and the campers come the next day. I want to make a difference, Lord. I remember when I was a camper thinking my camp counselors had it all together. Maybe they didn't have the world figured out, but they loved us still.

God, I am scared. Is it my fault that I feel distant from you? What am I doing wrong? My eating-disorder behaviors have been strong the past few days. As a result, my life has shrunk tremendously. I don't know what to say. I am pissed, God, and I feel that I am failing—failing in my relationship with you, with Chad, and with myself.

∞∞∞

It is so hard and frustrating. I am living about fifty feet from Chad and we're not talking. We are both trying to figure out whether we should take a break from dating each other. It seems so crazy. The past six months were so awesome. I had the time of my life. But to look at him now and see nothing like what I once did is scary. When he looks at me he must not see what he once did either. What seems to be real to me is not always fact. I don't know when everything between us began changing. I am deeply saddened that we have become so far removed from where we began that we don't know how to even carry on a conversation anymore.

⌒⌒

So it has been a long time since I wrote last. A week ago I got drunk. It never fails. When I drink I am much more vulnerable, and with my weakened inhibitions, I am likely to throw up. I did. Once a week we have a day off. Chad and I have spent only one of our days off together. This time he went with all these guys and some other girl counselors to Mexico. Well, he left without saying good-bye. He was just gone. It really hurt my feelings. Anyone deserves so much more. He has been talking to a couple of older counselors here about our relationship and what he should do with it. I think we both know what needs to be done, or at least I do.

We had this cookout with the campers and I had some chocolate cake, more than I thought I should. For the first time since I left Remuda, totally sober, I made myself throw up. I was so devastated. I could have delayed and not thrown up, but I just felt so bad inside. It was almost like it fit with the way I was feeling about myself. All this shit with Chad is killing me. I won't let go of the knowledge that if I were better things would be different, that I could make it all okay. If I weren't screwing up this would not be happening. I am so angry that I almost wanted to hurt myself, and I felt I deserved to be punished for not being more. Right before I did it, I remember being so angry and wanting it all to stop. I am just like every other bulimic in recovery. So much for my perfect record. I know my actions and feelings have so much more to do with my circumstance than my body. I am so angry with myself that I am not enough for Chad. Why can't I be better?

⌒⌒

I decided to make a change. I had been telling myself that my recovery came first, but obviously I have not been living as though this were true. One would think it would be obvious, but I didn't believe that I had not been listening to what I needed. After hitting what I consider to be a bottom in recovery, I decided I needed to take action. I was ready to give my talk in front of the camp, as many of the counselors do on the nights we have campfire. I talked about how God will never give us more than we can bear and that no matter how painful situations might become in our lives, he has a plan for all of us.

Here I was, telling all these kids exactly what I needed to hear. It left little justification for my actions only a few days ago. Great, so I was angry and in pain. God was there and I looked the other way. I had choices and I had many outs, but the bottom line is that I didn't have to throw up and I would have been able to cope just the same. As I was talking I began to feel like the person I love to live with. I had forgotten how much was inside to believe in. The room was filled with all the kids and I saw their innocent eyes as they hung on my every word, trying to understand, trying to see what they thought I knew to be true within myself. I guess I am not as grown up as I thought. But they looked at me and listened as though I had it all figured out. Then I looked at Chad and realized how lost I really was. How far would I let myself wander away from my heart, from this deeper vibration calling me back? In the instant I looked to him, I felt my confidence slip away. My eyes raced to focus on a row of little girls, all smiling. Their eyes were filled with love. I could see they loved me and that I didn't have to know the answers or live a flawless life for them to love me just the same. It was as though they didn't even think about life in terms of figuring it out. They just loved camp, loved their friends, and wanted nothing more than the present would give them.

This same night was Chad's first night back at camp since his long break in Mexico. I put the girls to bed and went down to his cabin. I had made up my mind that I had had enough. It wasn't just about deserving better treatment. I wanted more, and I knew that I much to gain in being alone. I respected this person so much and looked up to him in many ways. Now I was losing every bit of respect I had for him. I didn't want to see him the only way I was now accustomed to. We broke up by mutual agreement. We talked for about two hours. I felt great. I believe with all my heart that I did the best thing for myself and for him. I need to let him go. Within our silence I was losing myself and my feelings for him. Nothing is more important than my health. My slip and this experience are now history, and it can torture or teach.

Camp is good. I am very proud of myself. I have accomplished a lot. I have one week left; it is hard to believe.

⊂⊙〜⊙⊃

I am really excited! Dad came for parent's weekend. He has never been to TCU (except when he lived here). He was really great. We went to all the parties together and the football game. I loved his meeting all my friends and their parents. He is so funny. I had no idea that he was such a charmer. All my friends loved him.

Hanging out with him was strange. I almost felt as if it was someone else's dad I was getting to know as a real person. We had some good talks, since we were alone much of the time. As we were driving to breakfast Saturday morning I was reminded of a conversation we had almost a year ago. I was visiting him in LA, and we were making our usual trip to the garden store. I started asking him about his childhood and his parents. I have never seen him talk about his dad without his eyes filling or his voice cracking. I asked him whether he remembered his parents drinking and whether it bothered him. His face glazed over as he traveled back to his youth. There was a long silence before my father said softly, "I remember my parents' drinking. I would go around the house and pour out the alcohol. My father's drinking hurt me more than anything." As quickly as the memory came, it was gone, and he never spoke another word about it.

One of the things I love about my dad is that he can cry. I like seeing when something touches his heart and I can see how compassionate he is. The tears didn't come as I had assumed they would after what he shared with me. I didn't say a word—what could I say? Suddenly I felt sorry for my father not as he sat beside me at that moment, but as a boy—what must life have been like living with a father who drank enough to bring his grown son to tears? I knew for sure it was the first negative thing he had ever said about his dad to me. I will never forget that story.

I might be selfish for thinking this, but he was not the only one who was deeply hurt by a father's drinking. It was so apparent that the legacy was passed on. As a parent, he repeated the behavior that had probably pained him most as a child. If I had to name one thing that prohibited my dad and me from being close, without hesitation it would be his drinking and his resulting alcoholic personality. I have thought about that conversation many times, first with anger and then disgust, trying to justify and rationalize how he could repeat something that hurt him so much. I realized that I had actually received a gift that day, not some justification for a lifetime of resentments. He may never admit his mistake, the pain his drinking has caused, but by not forgiving him, in some way I become him, because I never grow to accept him.

⤙⤚

So many times I feel that I don't know who I am but that I am sure I know who other people are and what they need. I think I know more about fixing my family's and friends' feelings than my own. I know the right thing to say or the right thing to do. You would think coming to understand what I love and like would be straightforward.

Lasting change happens in infinitesimal increments. When you live the moments as they come, you never force them but accept them for what they are. When I smile deeply, I can feel it through my soul. That's what life is about: just living what is and allowing the mystery of life to sustain me. When I think about some of the happiest times, I am never happier than the morning after a good night out. When all the girls wake up, we leap into one of our small, twin beds. Then we tell the crazy stories, the events we lived through just hours before the sun rose. These talks are so motivating and enticing. We would rather die than miss the Sunday morning sequel. We laugh, fall on the floor, fighting for who can tell the next story. Each one in its unique way outdoes the others. I have the greatest friends in the world. I can't help but want to freeze those moments and soak them up so when I forget that I am lucky and blessed, I will remember all of us rolling on the floor fighting not to wet our pants. I swear the stories are priceless.

∞∞

I may not have the fairy tale I wish for, but I think I let go of a Snow White life when I stepped on the plane for Remuda. Writing is my refuge, the place where I can think everything bad. The dramas I carry on with myself and the mental mutiny I leave inside this book. The pages take a life of their own. Reading a book can change a person's life. Writing has guided my metamorphosis and helped me to endure it. It is by saying things in writing that I began to see. If I lived ten percent of what I fear, I would be dead. This is my saving grace and sowing of gratitude. Here I can for a moment live the demons, my greatest fears mixed with the worst thoughts. When I close this book, I can let it go and live the best and most authentic way I know. This is my sanctuary, the sanctuary of my heart and the truth I no longer want to live unconsciously.

∞∞

Heavenly Father, please hear me. I have run so far from my peace. I feel as though only a quarter of me exists consciously. I live out of fear and unrest. I trust nothing; nothing is right. I stare at my body, the beautiful one you gave me. I curse it, saying it is the source of my pain, my handicap, my greatest weakness. I even become ashamed and embarrassed, yes, for what I see when I look in the mirror, but even more, that I am in this place, this place of destruction and emptiness, entertaining these neurotic thoughts. How shallow and vain could my mind allow me to be? This is so much to bear. I constantly look to the mirror in final judgment. At times it holds the power to decide and reveal my destiny. In my mirror I see only the screw-ups, only the wrong. My body is an aesthetic object. No wonder I fear others' opinions of my body. If I objectify myself, I can't expect the world to do any better. A painting is beautiful, but in reality that is about the extent: it is an aesthetically pleasing object and for some offers a unique perspective. A person has infinite depth, but all my mirror sees is a messed up object. I pick at my skin, believing the pain I feel is deserved or even good for me. All my efforts are "less than" and inadequate. I find it hard to believe that any guy could find my body attractive when I'm more than a size four.

I know these lies far too well, but I seem to resist the truth nonetheless. The truth that would allow me a glimpse of hope feels far from my reach. I can ask myself, What is the truth? What do I know is true for me today, right here this very moment? I can tell myself I am not a size or a number, but that label in my skirt still holds more power than it was ever meant to hold. I am breathing, in recovery, healthy, and struggling well.

∞∞

John Holt and I were walking down the streets of New York when I finally got up the guts to ask him something only an honest guy could tell me. I casually said, "John Holt, do you think a guy would find my body attractive, or would I be more attractive to a guy if I were skinnier?" To no surprise he had the appropriate answer to my sick-minded question. "Whoever you end up with will love every part of you just like you are. There is not a body in the world that every guy will like, but whoever you are with will not see a body as an issue." Even though his words were honest, I wanted to hear either, "Chelsea you are absolutely perfect and I can't imagine a guy in the world not falling head over heels for you," or, "You fat little pig! Go lose some weight and you might have a chance." His answer was far too educated. He must have listened well at Remuda. He must really know me and love me.

∞∞

Things do change. By traveling to Austin last year I found myself on the doorstep of the house of a boy who would sweep me off my feet. Butterflies had filled my insides. It would be the biggest crush I had ever encountered. Not having a clue as to what lay ahead, I became all the more taken with him. I await- ed the next moment to come, as each held a new truth and understanding about who I was. That New Year's Eve could have sold as a screenplay. I thought I would melt after our first kiss, and I'll never consider the holiday overrated again. The previous year was too close to forget, making that night all the more important. One year ago I had been in bed by eight, wal- lowing in my addiction.

I find it comforting to remember the good as well as the bad, rather than a collection of permissible details. I realize the past no longer holds me captive and will hurt me if I continue to hold onto it. I guess the best part about dating Chad was that I lived for the moment, each moment as it should be. I learned the joy in the present. Every day was another day of life. He showed me that I could live my life differently, loving it more than I could have dreamed. For the next few months I lived in this fairy tale, leaving my life to chance and wanting not to control its course of action.

The Chad I knew then was not the same Chad I came to know that summer. I was not the same Chelsea either. We were both changing. I tell myself our breakup must have been right. I mean, I am not suppose to live in a mystical, carefree life for-ever, right? It's not realistic. But I was happy. I find myself won-dering why I could not have been more or been enough to make the fairy tale last. To all of our friends everything was per-fect, but obviously appearances don't tell the whole story. I have trouble letting the idea of us go. I pray, dear Lord, that in time I will let the beautiful past be just that, the beautiful past. I am grateful to know that fun, joy, and spontaneity really do exist outside of a Danielle Steele novel. I don't want to live in the fantasy of what could have been. If it had been meant to last, then it would have.

∽∾

I have not been doing well at all. It's like I have trained myself to see the worst. I work out three times a week, maybe four, and watch what I eat. I can tell I have lost some weight, three or four pounds maybe. I feel so responsible for everything in my life and the role I play in everyone else's. I am not will-ing to stop exercising. I don't think stopping would fix my problems. Yes, I am more body focused and have a need to horde food more. I am trying, or going to try, to spend more time with God. I really don't know where to go in my recovery. I just don't. I hate where I was, but I hate where I am. I can't believe, no, I won't let myself believe that this is the way my life is suppose to be. I am terrified because I strive for the answer, skipping the question entirely. Life has been nothing of what I thought it would be. So who knows what will turn it around? I have been here before. It's like I want to beat the crap out of God for not healing me. Maybe that is horrible and asking for too much, but I swear I feel like I have paid my dues.

∞∞

I am concerned. It is Friday night and I do not want to go out. It is convenient that my job takes up so much time and energy that I need to go to bed. I guess I am hiding behind it. When I want to be alone, ninety percent of the time it means I need to be with people. I need to confess that I have been throwing out my food. Or buying food and taking one bite and throwing it out the door. I will eat or covet the food even though I am not hungry. I wish I could understand the paradox of feeling lonely but still dreading the thought of going out. I don't get it. Things feel so normal and okay right now, but there must be something that is causing me to be so focused on my food.

∞∞

I never thought this would happen. (No, I am not going back to Remuda). Lauren and I are going to LA in about three hours for a spring break vacation at my dad's. I am scared as hell and yet really excited. I can tell my symptoms are flaring up. I give this trip to you, God, because I don't know how to balance the whole situation.

∞∞

For two years I have relinquished so many painful rituals, habits, and addictions. Today I find myself at the doorstep of most of them. Since my body has changed and I have lost a little weight, I have started riding the rollercoaster cycle. I tell myself I must keep up, maintain what I have achieved, do more. This serves as a distraction to every necessary bite I take. I do accept that I am running from something, and that something has made me really obsessive and neurotic. I am not being honest with myself. I am incredibly cranky, rigid in my routines, and frankly I would rather be alone. I would rather be righteous than happy. Basically I am frightened. This life casts a most enticing and alluring shadow. It is all lies. Why I still put this life on a pedestal I don't know. I am in pain and I don't want to live this life. God, please, I am begging you. Bless me with the courage to turn around and walk away, leaving this door closed. Please show me another way today. Never leave me. You are my life.

⟡⟡⟡

Father,

I am really scared, really scared. I look in the mirror and see only the image in front of me. I don't see me, I just can't. The body I am supposed to want is now appearing. The life I want is confused. The outside looks better, but my soul is so vulnerable—ready to embrace the lies. It creeps slowly, whispering, ultimately demanding, but always with grace. It trickles into my every breath and provides the backbone with which I stand, only to fall. My food is a big deal. I eat. I feel guilty. I tabulate, rationalize how I can stand to stay in my skin, how once again I can find a purpose to rise. Yes, I can build my wall higher and master its transparent presence. What is it that I won't admit? I am living the truth and I can't hide from myself. I am not doing well in recovery. I want to stop this now, but, but, but, what if, what if? Well what if I lose the body I have? What if I lose all I know today? Nothing frightens me more than losing hope, than losing my belief that I can live free from this bondage, this menacing shadow that resides within me. My failure is my fault. God, do you even know me? When you look at me, you must be disappointed. If I can't go to you, where am I to go? What is my purpose? I feel so burdened with the responsibility to know. I try to find a balance between exercise, food, and my body. I am just fucked up. With all my heart I ask you to please believe me. I do not want this disease. I don't want to walk each day knowing it is always a step ahead. Please, you must believe me, I don't want this. I want recovery with everything in my soul. What am I suppose to do, tell everyone that I am in trouble? Tell them all I am not doing well? What, and let them all down, make them lose all trust and faith in me? They can't help me. I know what they will say. I have heard all the psychobabble.

Lord, I don't get it. Just hit me in the head, fast. For now, I will just keep walking, walking the path I know feels horrible and is terrifying. But as promised, it will become part of my soul. It's not funny anymore. My hands are up and I am on my knees.

∞∞

A chapter in my life has come to a near close today.

Last Tuesday Ashley called. "Chelsea, I need to ask you something, but I am worried it will upset you."

In all confidence I said, "No, go ahead, it won't."

She continued, "One of my best friends, Suzanne, knows Michael's brother, David. David and his wife have a one-year-old little boy. I am really concerned and I thought you would want to know that they innocently leave their child in Michael's care sometimes." All too quickly I was four years old again. My little-girl thoughts of a dirty, mean, and gross man were spinning. Me lying on his basement floor bed was an image I could not shut out. As quickly as the memories came back, it made that day all the more haunting. Not revealing the chills of fear his name alone still sent through my heart, I continued, "Wait, you mean to tell me you know where Michael is? He has a wife and a child of his own now? This is the most hideous thing I have ever heard. That sick bastard. How can his wife not know? I want to tell her. She has got to know!

"Ashley, what can I do? David and his wife need to know the truth. I know David has to know what happened to me. I remember him never wanting me to go play with Michael or to stay in his room. He has to know."

Ashley said, "I have thought about the best way to tell his wife, and I think Suzanne wants to invite David's wife over for their kids to play and then have you come over to tell her."

Calmly, she continued, "Chelsea, I think that would be great if you told Michael's wife, but why not start with his sister-in-law? She would be the more willing to accept or even hear what you have to say."

"Fine, set the whole thing up and I will do whatever I need to. I just can't believe this. Let me know what time and where."

"Okay, I will call Suzanne," Ashley promised.

"Hey, Ashley thanks. And thank you for being so protective of my feelings and realizing this is a delicate subject, but I am really okay with it all now."

Thirty minutes later the phone rang. It was Suzanne. She assured me that I was making the right decision and that they (David and his wife) needed to know.

With everything in me and everything positive I could pray for, I drove to Suzanne's that Tuesday. A navy Altima arrived at the same time. A dark-haired woman and her little boy got out of that car. All I could think of was what I knew and what she was going to find out. Confidently I introduced myself. I couldn't help staring at this baby boy, wondering whether what I was about to tell would really matter or whether his mother would even listen. Keeping my eyes fixed on him, along with the truth, was my greatest source of strength. We rang the door bell. Everything was in slow motion except my mind. With all my heart I knew this had to be done.

Suzanne got the children playing in another room. She came in and sat down next to Melissa, explaining my purpose. "Chelsea is here because there are some things you need to know."

All this time I was staring at the carpet, praying I wouldn't pass out. I was terrified. Here I was about to tell this newlywed, with her new baby, that she married a man whose brother they all love is a child molester. How welcome could this be? I had been in enough counseling and had adequate social skills to know I had to look her in the face. Moreover, I had nothing to be ashamed of and no longer did I have to hide. I took a deep breath, praying with everything in me that God would be there and give me the strength. I raised my eyes as the first word fell out, relinquishing much of the fear.

"Melissa, I want you to know that you can ask me anything. I will elaborate on anything, and I will do what I can to help you and your little boy. I am hear today because of your brother-in-law, Michael. When I was four years old. . ." Her eyes never moved from her blank stare at my mouth. The more I told, the more honest and real I was to myself, God, and with the thought of every child he had touched and would touch, the words came easier, but always they came in love. Her shock was not a surprise, but I was stunned at her willingness to accept the painful truth, and even more, at her desire for me to tell her husband, David. All I could think then was Michael's brother, Michael's brother whom I had not spoken to in at least twelve years. She wanted this, and painfully I knew I needed this. In reality, despite my fear, I wanted to tell David the truth.

Melissa decided the best thing was for her to tell David before I came over. After much deliberation, she decided tomorrow night at 6:30. That would give him enough time to come in from work, put the baby to sleep, and enough time for Melissa to brief him on my purpose.

∞

Six o'clock is approaching, and I am becoming more and more anxious and scared. I called Melissa early this morning to let her know that I had decided I wanted my mom with me. She also felt her being there would be good. I agree, considering that mom knows most of what I know and some things I don't. I know I appear brave on the outside, but I am dying. I feel like a child again. I know in my heart what I will tell them may not change anything. They may not even believe me. I know what happened is true, and telling them is one way I can make a right out of a life-changing wrong. The thought of my fear causing their little boy or any other child to be sexually abused is a weight I could not live with.

∞

God, please be with me, please be with me, PLEASE, PLEASE, was the only thing I could sanely think as Mom and I waited for the door to open. I never asked how to say it. There was nothing pretty about this truth. I didn't want to rehearse anything, not even their reaction. Thinking of what might come would only cripple me. I just wanted God to show me at the very moment. I took a deep, shaking breath as I heard his hand on the door. Mom looked at me. There was nothing to say now. We both knew what we had to do. David and Melissa asked us to sit down. Mom was sociably correct in her small talk. His eyes were red—the result of tears I assumed. His face was stark and white. The house seemed gravely quiet. I had nothing to say. I had yet to make eye contact with him, fearing that when I did I would see Michael's eyes, the ones I had tried to forget all these years. I knew that he knew something now, but I wasn't sure to what degree.

"David, I know this must not be easy for you," Mom said.

"Yeah." His head hung, eyes staring at the floor. Seated in a chair at arm's reach from the couch Mom and I delicately rested on, he quietly said, "I am so confused. Will you tell me? I don't understand. Tell me." He was shaking his head.

Everything went numb—my hands, my feet. Everything in the room disappeared but David and his question. Staring at the top of his curly head, I decided I had one shot and that I wanted him to know what happened that day—every last detail.

"I had been playing at Mimi's house. It was about three in the afternoon, a little before Mom routinely came from work to get me. Like any other day all the kids were outside playing. I had been in your yard playing with your dog. Your mom came to the door and asked me some questions and then she said, "Michael wants to see you downstairs in his room." I remember walking down the stairs to his basement room. They were covered in multicolored shag carpet. There was a wooden railing on the side that I used, because the stairs were steep. It was dark except for the light in Michael's room. The door was open and I stood just inside the door. He didn't say much, except that he wouldn't hurt me. He picked me up and laid me on his big bed. It had an itchy bedspread. I was wearing one of my favorite dresses, blue with a lace collar and white polka dots. As always I was wearing my Lollipop underwear with "Chelsea" monogrammed across the bottom. He lifted my dress up to where the hem was at my neck. He opened my legs up, pushing my knees where they were bent. I remember he took off his underwear and I saw his brown pubic hair. Then I looked to my left, into the bathroom, staring at the baby blue tile-covered walls. He turned my head toward him, placing a washcloth over my eyes. I felt something touching me, rubbing me, and then he let me see his penis run up and down my vagina. I don't know how long I had been down there when his mom called from the top of the stairs, "Michael, Chelsea needs to go now. Her mom is here." Michael jumped off the bed and I ran up from the dark. My feet suddenly seemed less solid. They stumbled on a few of the steep stairs, going as fast as they could carry me. I remember telling my mom something after that, and then that's all I remember."

Then Mom talked for a little while about what I told her and how she told John Holt and Ashley. She related how she contacted the "experts" and how they said not to make a big deal out of it because I was so young that they hoped I would just forget. As she told David what had happened, I was reminded of the routine we followed for about two years following the incident. Each day as we passed Michael's house on the way to Mimi's, Mom would say, "There is that mean Michael, that bad Michael. We don't like him." Then I would say, "I don't like him. He is mean and he is bad."

While Mom was talking, I had a chance to really look at David without his noticing. I was surprised that his face remained empty, like we were telling him something that had no relevance in his life, much less something that went on in his own house.

With the same emotionless expression he said to me, "I mean, was this something that you thought about sometimes or . . . ?"

Up to this point I was really strong. Everything I had told him were details that I had worked through, cried over, starved over, thrown up over. But no one—all the therapists, my family, or even myself—had asked that question. I knew without hesitation as tears filled my eyes that I had to explain.

"That happened to me when I was four. After that day I had no concept of a life without that room haunting my every thought. I knew all had changed. I knew by what had happened I would never be the same. At first I was not ashamed. I didn't even think about it being my fault. As time passed, the silence and the secret, my secret, cultivated shame. Every morning, every day, I prayed the same prayer, 'God please let them all forget. Please don't let them think I am a dirty, bad girl. Please today, Lord, help me feel normal.' I remember one time specifically when I was in the fourth grade. I was walking down the hall at school with a group of girls, 'the cool girls,' and thinking in the midst of our laughing and comparing our new Swatch Watches, 'I am not like you. I am so different. I am tarnished, messed up, and bad. I had this credence that I was this dark, blackened child who could never be like them. Pure, carefree, and innocent were things I would never be because I was different. If they only knew how gross and bad I was on the inside, they would think I was a freak. So to answer your question, did I think about this every day? Yes, I didn't know anything else. It has taken me a long time to get to the point where I can sit across from Michael's brother and tell you what happened. I would not have come unless I knew in my heart that it was never my fault. At four years old I was a child—a victim. Today I am not. This is one of many ways I can show myself, you, your family, and mine that I will walk on—continuing to make the most out of a hideous, disgusting, and life-changing event. I have given you all the information I know. I want more than anything for your son and Michael's child to be safe, but that is now out of my control. What I want from this is to give Michael and your entire family his poison back. It's not mine. It never was meant to be mine, and I am not responsible for his sins. I will be damned if I let him have one more day of my life or pain my family with his sickness. I am no longer a victim and no longer does that day haunt me. Mom, I am ready to go."

I hadn't anticipated much about this meeting, but when David got up from his chair, apologizing for his brother and hugging Mom, I thought I had done it. The challenge was over. 'What if he tries to hug me?' I thought. It seemed like the worst thing that could possibly happen at that moment. His appearance was still enough like Michael to make my stomach churn, and as he leaned toward me I thought, 'My God, how can I hug this man who for me is the closest I will ever come to Michael?' And yet I knew it was the best way to truly make peace with this demon of fear. When I hugged him, I meant it. I meant that I was grateful he could listen and empathize, and that Mom and I could walk away holding hands—hands that were more free than they had been in sixteen years.

She pulled our car around the corner and stopped. I began to wail, crying the deepest tears, deep as I had ever known. These tears were healing tears, sealing the darkest scars and quieting my greatest fears. She said nothing as she held me, not a sound. I felt something for Michael in separateness that I hadn't when I held him in my life. It was forgiveness, yes, but it was something more. It was very close to love for him as a human. I cried and cried, and for once in my life, I was truly free. I will never pass his house without thinking, at least for a moment, that today was a fulfillment of my wish.

⊙⊙

The darkness I felt inside for so many years existed without my realizing its crippling effect. The more I seek to understand its presence, the more I understand the relevance of the act of bingeing and the pain of purging. For whatever reason, the action of sticking my fingers down my throat repeatedly, over and over, bringing the food up in my hands, then throwing it down in the toilet, flushing it away, somehow made me feel like I could reach the pain, the misunderstood and misplaced darkness. I felt I deserved to hurt. The insides were all bad, dirty, nasty, and weird. What I did to myself seemed only fitting for what I knew was looming beneath what we all saw. Obviously I would do anything to take the darkness into the light. I wanted to stop hiding, stop running from the poison that consumed me. My futile attempt to make the outside perfect caused an immeasurable amount of pressure. I held my breath in the hope that it would work, that I could make the outside so right it would change the inside back to clean or normal.

My cunning plan to achieve perfection was never meant to last. Anyone knows a person with an eating disorder dies from it, recovers from it, or at worst, lives out her whole life in an isolated, empty, baffling obsession. She can see the light but never dares to rise to the challenge of living with truth and life on its terms.

I don't attribute my eating disorder to one thing. Remuda taught us there are many logs on the fire. I do believe that the sexual abuse was a big log for me. It's hard to say to how great an extent it contributed to my eating disorder. In reality its magnitude is irrelevant. Recognizing and working through the pieces, the logs on the fire, is my primary concern.

∽∾

It is a terrifying thing not trusting yourself. I have known for a couple of months that I'd been accepted to a college program to study in London for a semester. In addition to taking a course on art history (held at the National Gallery) and a course on musical theater, I will have an internship with the NBC foreign news bureau. This is so great, but I am scared to death. I am finally getting the chance to really go away, far from where I live life. However, I want no set plan or way to do anything.

Well, I can't get this image out of my head. I see myself getting off the plane and the next thing I know I am on some random street in London flailing around like a fish out of water. As soon as I was old enough to learn about independence, look what I chose for myself—an eating disorder. Now I am scared to death that I will do it again. Not trusting yourself to be able to take care of yourself is far from encouraging. This is one of those times when I just need to do it: get on that plane and trust that with God's help I can do this. I mean, why even get into recovery if I won't let myself live opportunities like this?

∞∞

I can't help but fear that my attraction to regular exercising is a behavior that hurts me, something I do because I don't know how to cope or deal with the other issues. Maybe I can't put my finger on the cause right now, but I tell myself it has nothing to do with normal fears like being in Europe in a completely new environment with new people and a different culture. Rather, I fear it has to do with the body I know now and the one I might develop while I am there. I don't like writing that I am scared or that I have been running for the past three days trying to understand where to go or what to do with this fear. Going to Europe for a semester will be enough of a challenge. I don't need to make the transition any more difficult. I can tell myself how horrible I am and how much I am screwing up, but it does not help. As a matter of fact it intensifies the whole matter. Those thoughts drive me further from my heart, where innocently, quietly, and patiently, the answer lies. It waits without condemnation and without being tainted by emotions, ripe and ready to be woven into this huge tapestry. I am so busy running from my pain—or more simply, from what exists. To just accept my truth as a matter of fact, as a matter of life, would be much simpler.

Today will be the beginning of the fulfillment of one of my greatest dreams. I am going to live in London for five months. I know in my heart I am ready. Being too afraid to go because of my recovery would defeat all my hopes for recovery, its primary motive: to be free so that I can live and I can learn. To stay home because I am scared would be a great hindrance to my success in recovery.

I would be lying to say I wasn't scared, scared of the newness, scared of the drive that propels me to push, scared of the intensity that fuels so much of my emotion, and scared of myself. I have no control. The desire is so strong. I know the steps, but I find my feet walking differently. I am sorry I am my greatest enemy. I won't do this alone, but with all my heart open to you, God. I know this adventure is right.

This is my major separation, a chance to form a life for myself, build a new framework. I don't want this chaos built on the instability and insanity of an addiction. I don't need it anymore. I am not an extension of my eating disorder.

∞∞

I couldn't sleep for my thoughts and obsessive thinking. Perhaps the obsessive thinking is the one thing that I can make sure won't change. It is familiar. Tonight, these thoughts are not nagging and painful as they normally are but are almost a peaceful refuge for the unfamiliarity of my surroundings. The majority live the challenge and strive to learn and grow. The others must be scared, alone, afraid, and terrified of this big world I have not yet come to know. This world does not look or feel safe. Maybe a part of me doubts my ability to take care of myself now, but I will. I will, and the addiction won't. It may feel scary to live here, but I will make choices as the person I know now, not as the sick one. Yes, it is scary, but the other is deadly. If anything will suck the life out of me, it will. It has and it can do it again. This is serious. My fear and uncertainty are real, but I know a different way.

⊙⊙

### In London

I call home and it is all the same, everyone is the same. My family is still talking about the same stuff, the same insignificant troubles. I get sucked right back into all their problems. I have been gone almost two months and I hardly call home, but when I do, it's like they have stored up all this stuff to unload. I have to fake a bad connection just so I can get off. One of the greatest gifts of being here is that I am an ocean away, so I can't feel responsible for anything that goes on. I am glad I am not there to hear all the day-to-day "tragedies." I hang up the phone and I am gasping for air. I am tense, my chest is tight, and I am on edge by the time our conversation ends. I struggle to think straight. To see as I did before my thoughts instinctively returned home. I do not want to go home. I have it so good here. Damn, it really kills me that what I remember about my life at home, what I long to embrace, has not changed like I think. Too often, my mind removes all the bad from the memories, leaving only the good. In fact, I see my past refuge much differently now that I am removed from it. They are still the same, which is fine, but I am not satisfied with my remaining stagnant. They still react just the same. I am going to let go of them and live life up while I am here. They can't touch me. "I am an ocean away, an ocean away, and ocean away. . ." and I want to relish in that.

Remuda talked about how the world I left will not have changed upon my return, even though I will have. They challenged me to recognize what action I will take to maintain sanity within the same context in which I got sick. At the time I don't think I was consciously in a position to acknowledge the scary familiarity of my once unhealthy surroundings. Now in retrospect I can see how I lock right back in the mold. It is fascinating how much my world has changed in just two months, but the world I separated from has not skipped a beat. I just step out. Since I lived in it, seeing my life realistically was impossible because I saw it through the same eyes. I almost don't want to return, not to the way I lived in the world I left. I am in no way blaming anyone for not changing from my perspective, but I am confronted with the reality that I will return. Being here, I often find myself thinking what I want to choose for my life, what I want to inhabit from here, and what I want to keep with me. How will I reshape a life that already has a form-fitting mold, which for the most part has worked and awaits to embrace me?

I am truly amazed that I have been fine, in fact thrived, without my ritual recovery patterns. I am not advocating absence from therapy, but God is really taking care of me.

When I think back, my need to leave home, to go to London, seems almost inevitable. I have always wanted to know a life on my own. The thought of separating from my family has always intrigued me. I found peace in knowing that someday I would live out the experience or face the repercussions of not honoring my intuition.

For as long as I can remember I have had this feeling that I need to leave home. It was hard for me to explain, but I've known I needed to go far away, where I could forget about Fort Worth, my family, and all the stuff that has made me into who I am—all my self-assigned responsibilities, the daily family ordeals, the life I had come to know so well. Leaving was never about running away or running from my problems. I've just had this feeling that inside of me were things I want to know and want to live. I know that my eyes are so sheltered. I still have much to explore and learn. Within myself I want to live the things that I am not even conscious of. Time will separate me from my life then and my thoughts now. By staying where I knew I would always be safe, I would never grow. It is true that after being in another country, being far away for awhile, I see things in a different way. I now know that it will be impossible to return unchanged. I have this peace that whatever I do or wherever I go, I will be fine. I know this experience will always be a sanctuary from my doubts in my ability to take care of myself.

∽⊙∽

In my young life it is hard to say that one year is more important than another. But the two and a half years in my eating disorder and the one building up (to total three and a half) were monumental. Any chunk of your life devoted to or fixated on one goal, is bound to have an impact on the whole. From fifteen to eighteen was a time for my friends to separate from their parents, make mistakes, make bad choices, and not really care about much but going out and dating. Somewhere in the midst of the chaos, they learned and figured out how to take care of themselves and start making decisions for their lives, understanding their needs and how to meet them. I took a very different road, devoting my heart and ultimately my soul to slowly destroying my confidence and independence.

In all, I missed out. I knew that to some extent at the time. When I entered recovery, I had a deeper understanding of how shallow, dark, and alone my life really was. Not until today had I realized how much confidence I had lost in my ability to take care of myself, my internal instinct to identify my needs and know how to meet them. Being in a foreign country and totally alone, I can't recall when I have felt so content. See, when my peers were learning, I was hiding—from what I don't know. But when the time came for me to choose and I had the gradual freedom of privileges with age, I chose differently. I was learning, teaching, and choosing to kill myself. I chose to starve and to throw up. There is no confidence or self-esteem in either act. I wasn't building a foundation but pouring quicksand. No wonder I was scared out of my mind to come to London. Considering the choices I had already made, it was hard to have trust in myself and my own understanding. Like everyone, I was given the chance, the time naturally designed for building independence and to grow. I chose to live through an eating disorder. I chose to abuse my body in the most painful way.

I believe now in something I didn't know was there. Something was lacking in my recovery. It was knowing I can take care of myself and make healthy choices for myself, not because they know what is right for me or what I "should" do, but because I now know. Only I know what is right for me. I believe in myself and my ability to be self-sufficient. I guess it has taken me longer to learn about the strong and capable me. The gratitude I feel is immense. It doesn't seem to matter whether or not you know at a young age that life is difficult, because eventually you will learn.

# The Road to Recovery

*I*f there is repetition here, it is because I have not read Chelsea's journal, and I do not know how much she has chosen to share. It is her decision and her story. What I am committed to share is my part in her story so that family members of a person with an eating disorder can learn from my mistakes and consider some of the solutions I found for myself. As I am sure you are learning, eating disorders are extremely complicated and there are no quick remedies. Before Chelsea returned from her brief stay at boarding school, I had begun reading the first of many books and articles I was to read over the next year. Gaining education and knowledge are my first suggestions for family members and friends of someone with an eating disorder.

I focused on Chelsea's recovery for the next year. With her father's help we located a wonderful therapist. Chelsea seemed to be working hard at beating the disease. Regrettably, when she conquered bulimia she replaced it with anorexia. As her pounds began to fall off, I observed intently as if watching would keep her well. Of course I tried to camouflage my hyper-vigilance. I never made comments about how little she ate or what she did not choose to put on her plate. Looking back at my futile attempts to protect her, I see I was like a mother obsessed with sudden infant death syndrome who stands by her sleeping *baby's crib at night, counting her baby's breaths. Like that mother I was exhausted from watching and worrying. I also wasn't sleeping. At night my fears were monstrous. What if she did not get well? I would try to think of the right thing to say, the right thing to cook, the right way to act. Nothing was working. Chelsea continued to starve.*

*I tried to cook low-fat healthy food. I read and prepared recipes that promised flavor without fat. Chelsea joined me in the "healthy" cooking. She wanted to go to the grocery store with me and liked to go daily. Ironically our relationship seemed to revolve around food. Eating out was awful. As she became more isolated from friends and social interaction, I enabled her by answering the telephone and taking messages. I eventually became exasperated with her rarely returning the messages I took for her.*

*Amazingly my marriage survived my obsession with being there for Chelsea in case she needed me. Bill was patient, sympathetic, and loving. He had been like a father to Chelsea since she was about two years old. Bill was frustrated with the disease no one could make sense of. He seemed to be able to separate his loving feelings for Chelsea from her eating disorder. He would go to whatever restaurant she chose, help the waiter understand that she did not want any butter or oil on her steamed vegetable, and then be the one to send it back if she detected any trace of the forbidden coating.*

*Frozen fat-free yogurt had become a staple. I enabled her by driving to the closest yogurt shop, which was not close, anytime she requested it. The time or inconvenience I never considered, only that she was eating something. Looking back, I realize this insanity was right up there with my going to aerobics classes with her. It was so painful to watch her pushing herself on the highest stack of steps, working her arms as her spindly legs pounded up and down to burn the maximum calo-*

ries. It was so distressing to be there, but I was afraid to not be there. She seemed to need me there so that is where I had to be.

My friends were so supportive. They called, listened, prayed, wept, and laughed with me. Some understood more than others because they had struggled with daughters who had eating disorders. Frequently they would refrain from asking about Chelsea by asking what I was doing to take care of myself. My replay was something like, "Oh, I'm doing fine." They knew better because they knew me. One of my oldest friends took me on a long weekend to Santa Fe. I thought she did not know about Chelsea because she no longer lived in Fort Worth. I never asked her, but I am convinced that she was reaching out with love to be there for me and to give me a break from the disease.

After I had spent a year of futile attempts to be the perfect mother of a daughter who was starving, a friend asked me again what I was doing for myself. She asked me if I would like to go to an Alanon meeting with her. Alanon is a twelve-step program for relatives or friends of an alcoholic. Certainly Chelsea was not an alcoholic, but I had learned that an eating disorder was like an addiction. My friend said attending Alanon had really helped her and wisely suggested that during the Alanon meeting whenever I heard the word "alcoholic" I should mentally substitute "eating disordered."

I don't know why I agreed to go with her the next morning, but once the meeting started I knew that it was right where I needed to be. Tears rolled down my cheeks throughout the hour meeting. The topic they were discussing was "Letting go and letting God." It was a solution I had never considered, because I thought I had to take care of Chelsea, be in charge of her recovery, and giver her the support she needed. I heard at the meeting that morning that the first step was to admit, that I was powerless over her disease. It was a truth I had not been *willing to admit because my greatest fear was that if I gave up, she would die. Combating her disease had become my addiction, my disease.*

*I made a commitment to myself to attend at least five more meetings before deciding if Alanon was helpful to me. I can't describe the sense of peace I felt in those meetings as I heard others share their experience, strength, and hope. I continued to attend Alanon and still do today. This twelve-step program has made all the difference in my sanity, my marriage, my relationship with God and family, and especially in my response to Chelsea and her eating disorder. It is not a program for everyone, but it was a lifesaver to me. It continues to help me live a positive and balanced life one day at a time.*

*I had been attending several Alanon meetings each week for about six months, when one night Chelsea told me she thought she needed to go to a residential treatment center. I will not go into the numerous conversations we had that night or in the days that followed other than to say she confessed that she was not just anorexic but had relapsed into bulimia as well. As we waited for her departure for treatment at Remuda Ranch and during her weeks there, I would put myself to sleep at night repeating the Serenity Prayer from Alcoholics Anonymous: "God grant me the serenity to accept the things I cannot change, the courage to change the things I can, and the wisdom to know the difference."*

*The thought of my daughter living at a treatment center in another state at first terrified me. But I had learned in Alanon to let go and let God. I had also come to understand that I did not have to have all the answers for Chelsea and that not knowing what would help her did not mean I was a failure as a mother. Allowing her to make decisions and choices for herself without my advice was a way of empowering her to be responsible for her health. Once she was there I felt a deep sense of relief that she was right where she needed to be, where she was supposed to be. Our brief scheduled telephone calls were tearful but reassuring. I heard renewed strength in her voice, as well as hope and determination to beat the disease. Bill and I celebrated when she told us that she was now enjoying some of her "forbidden" foods she had not eaten in a year. The time seemed to pass quickly for us, although I imagine it seemed much longer for her. It was already time for us to go for family week, and we could not wait to see the daughter we felt we had lost.*

*I will not detail family week, but I will speak in general to my experience at Remuda Ranch. From the moment we arrived I felt even better about the staff and their multidisciplinary approach. It was a setting full of love, acceptance, and wisdom. I learned even more about eating disorders and especially how twelve-step programs such as Alanon were the best places that I could find the support and skills I needed to relate to Chelsea. I gained more insight into myself and our family dynamics. We were guided to share truth and love and it worked wonders for me as I believe it did for all of us. I was so proud of Chelsea. I was so proud of our family.*

*Chelsea came home about two weeks later. Her reentry into our home was not totally smooth, but amazingly, it was not the difficult adjustment I feared. I walked on eggshells only the first few hours. She was so grounded in her recovery that she reassured me daily, not in words but in attitude and action, of her determination to stay healthy, happy, and free of disease. Remuda's professional staff warned and prepared us for the minor or major relapses that always occur. Thank goodness she was now in charge of her recovery; I just tried to stay out of her way. I had learned not to be hypervigilant. What a gift! I felt better and better each day as her graduation from high school quickly approached and the time for her to leave for college arrived.*

*Today I am so grateful for Chelsea's amazing recovery. We have our happy, healthy Chelsea back. But I am also grateful for what I hated the most—her disease. It is hard to imagine that I could be grateful for something that caused such pain and anguish, for something that almost killed her. But her disease helped all of us grow and learn more about ourselves. All of our relationships improved. All of us can experience strength, hope, and love in a way we did not even know was possible. Her disease and recovery gave us an incredible life-changing experience. My gratitude list keeps growing daily. The miracles were always there. Now I just see them.*

# Epilogue

The events of these years that I write about are not unique to my experience. In fact, they are far too common. For me to see the truth, I had to say it first. Writing was my voice. I wrote out of need. I did not transcribe my journal into a book to glorify myself or sell my story. Many times I cringed at the thought of my most intimate secrets being exposed. What kept me going is the hope that in these pages someone might gain insight, hope, or understanding. I wish that I could prevent any woman or girl from falling into this bottomless pit or hug every mother and father, telling them, "She'll be okay." I hope the one thing you gain from reading my journal is that a person suffering from an eating disorder must want to live and do whatever it takes. You can't do it for her. As for readers struggling with eating disorders themselves, maybe this example will shorten the days of denial or will let you know that you are not alone. My motivation to reveal everything I wrote was only there because of God. I write this for him. He is the reason I share this story that is without an end.